Oral Precancer

Oral Precancer

Diagnosis and Management of Potentially Malignant Disorders

Edited by

Peter Thomson

BDS MBBS MSc PhD FDSRCS(Eng) FFDRCS(Irel) FRCS(Ed)

Professor of Oral and Maxillofacial Surgery, Newcastle University

Honorary Consultant Oral and Maxillofacial Surgeon
Newcastle upon Tyne Hospitals NHS Foundation Trust

Newcastle upon Tyne, UK

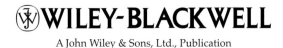
A John Wiley & Sons, Ltd., Publication

This edition first published 2012 © 2012 by John Wiley & Sons, Ltd.

Blackwell Publishing was acquired by John Wiley & Sons in February 2007. Blackwell's publishing program has been merged with Wiley's global Scientific, Technical and Medical business to form Wiley-Blackwell.

Registered office: John Wiley & Sons, Ltd, The Atrium, Southern Gate, Chichester, West Sussex, PO19 8SQ, UK

Editorial offices: 9600 Garsington Road, Oxford, OX4 2DQ, UK
The Atrium, Southern Gate, Chichester, West Sussex, PO19 8SQ, UK
111 River Street, Hoboken, NJ 07030-5774, USA

For details of our global editorial offices, for customer services and for information about how to apply for permission to reuse the copyright material in this book please see our website at www.wiley.com/wiley-blackwell.

The right of the author to be identified as the author of this work has been asserted in accordance with the UK Copyright, Designs and Patents Act 1988.

Library of Congress Cataloging-in-Publication Data

A catalogue record for this book is available from the British Library.

Wiley also publishes its books in a variety of electronic formats. Some content that appears in print may not be available in electronic books.

Set in 10.5/13pt Sabon by Thomson Digital, Noida, India
Printed and bound in Singapore by Markono Print Media Pte Ltd

1 2012

Contents

List of Contributors

Dr Michaela L. Goodson BMedSci BDS MBBS MFDSRCS MRCS
Specialist Registrar in Oral and Maxillofacial Surgery, Northern Deanery
Honorary Clinical Lecturer, Newcastle University, Newcastle upon Tyne, UK

Dr C. Max Robinson BDS MSc PhD FDSRCS FRCPath
Senior Lecturer in Oral Pathology, Newcastle University
Honorary Consultant Pathologist, Newcastle upon Tyne Hospitals NHS
Foundation Trust, Newcastle upon Tyne, UK

Professor Philip Sloan BDS PhD FDSRCS FRCPath
Consultant Pathologist, Newcastle upon Tyne Hospitals NHS
Foundation Trust
Honorary Professor, Newcastle University, Newcastle upon Tyne, UK

Peter Thomson BDS MBBS MSc PhD FDSRCS(Eng) FFDRCS(Irel) FRCS(Ed)
Professor of Oral and Maxillofacial Surgery, Newcastle University
Honorary Consultant Oral and Maxillofacial Surgeon, Newcastle upon Tyne
Hospitals NHS Foundation Trust, Newcastle upon Tyne, UK

Preface

This book has its origins some 30 years ago during my experiences as a dental undergraduate student attending specialist oral surgery and oral medicine clinics at a prestigious dental teaching hospital in northwest England in the early 1980s. I was fascinated to observe the number and variety of patients who presented with white and/or red oral mucosal lesions and to learn of their varied aetiologies, histopathological diagnoses and, perhaps most significantly of all, to discover their potential high risk for transformation to mouth cancer.

My early interest and enthusiasm to study this beguiling spectrum of oral precancer disease, however, quickly became tempered by the realisation that my clinical teachers, many of whom were senior clinicians and professors of international repute, were unable to determine the individual risk of patients undergoing carcinogenesis. Nor could they offer a reliable prognosis for disease progression or apparently any appropriate treatment intervention. Perhaps worst of all was to actually encounter those unfortunate patients who, despite regular clinic attendance for examination and reassurance, subsequently went on to develop oral cancer.

During my professional career, I have been extremely fortunate to have had the opportunity to continue this personal interest in oral oncology and to have been able to pursue a number of studies into the scientific basis of oral cancer and precancer diagnosis and management. As I commenced my clinical training, firstly within hospital dentistry, then medical undergraduate studies, followed by a period of research work in the field of oral epithelial biology before ultimately specialising as an oral and maxillofacial surgeon, I learned a great deal more about the devastating consequences, both in terms of morbidity and mortality, of invasive squamous cell carcinoma of the oral cavity.

Today oral cancer remains a lethal disease, with a near 50% mortality at 5 years. The consequences of that disease process and the application of the primary treatment modalities of tumour resection and/or chemoradiotherapy produce significant and distressing morbidities, in terms of a loss of form and function, to both the mouth and the face for those patients who survive their cancer treatment. Unfortunately, these problems are growing rather than lessening in significance. Worldwide, the annual mortality rates from mouth and oropharyngeal cancers are expected to rise from 370 000 to nearly 600 000 a year by 2030. This emphasises the seriousness of the disease as a truly global health problem. Some authors have even predicted that we will, in effect, actually experience a worldwide epidemic of oral cancer during the latter part of the 21st century.

It is important to stress, however, that it is not my intention to write a book about oral cancer. Indeed, there are many excellent textbooks available that encompass all the aetiology, diagnosis and management of mouth cancer that the interested reader may require. Rather, this book focuses upon oral precancer – that clinically recognisable state composed of a variety of distinct oral lesions or sometimes more widespread conditions, which is now more commonly referred to collectively as potentially malignant disorders, that may precede the development of invasive squamous cell carcinoma of the oral cavity.

Potentially malignant disorders therefore offer clinicians a potential therapeutic window of opportunity to intervene and to attempt to halt the progress of oral mucosal disease before the onset of irreversible carcinogenesis.

Unfortunately, there remains significant controversy over the efficacy of interventional therapies in preventing cancer and there are thus no universally agreed treatment protocols for oral precancer lesions. Whilst a vast literature of published papers on potentially malignant disease has accrued through the years, quite literally numbering many thousands, there remains substantial confusion in their overall purpose, their use of terminology and the conclusions that they draw. Perhaps most frustratingly of all, this body of literature provides virtually no consensus on how to coordinate treatment or provide clinical care for precancer patients.

The principal aim in writing this book, therefore, is to propose a rational basis for an interventional clinical management protocol. This is based upon several years of observational clinical research and patient cohort treatment studies, all of which have been designed with the specific intent of trying to prevent potentially malignant disorders progressing to oral cancer.

I have not attempted in this book to construct a comprehensive worldwide literature review and critique. This is because, quite frankly, no consensus view could be extrapolated from such an exercise but also because such a work would be highly unreadable and it would fail in my attempt to deliver a concise summary of our current understanding of the nature and behaviour of oral potentially malignant disorders. I have, however, listed many contemporaneous review articles in the reference sections that accompany each chapter, to allow the researcher who wishes to pursue aspects of this work in more detail to be able to do so.

Like most clinicians, I owe an enormous personal debt to my many clinical teachers and surgical trainers through the years, but I particularly wish to acknowledge and thank all my patients for their stoicism and loyalty and especially the trust they have bestowed on me as both their advisor and surgeon. It is for them, and future patients like them, that I have written this book.

Peter Thomson
Newcastle upon Tyne, UK
2011

Acknowledgements

I would like to acknowledge the important contributions of my expert co-authors Michaela Goodson, Max Robinson and Philip Sloan for their help and active involvement in producing this book. Without them, this manuscript would undoubtedly have been much poorer and only a pale shadow of its current form. I also wish to thank my postgraduate students who, with their boundless intelligence and ceaseless enthusiasm have, over the years, encouraged and stimulated my research into the scientific basis of oral carcinogenesis. Ultimately this has helped develop the approach to the diagnosis and management of oral potentially malignant disorders presented in this book. I especially wish to mention in this regard Omar Hamadah, Ameena Diajil, Rachel Green and Michaela Goodson. Much of their individual contributions to the scientific development of oral precancer research is presented and acknowledged in this work.

I would also like to express my thanks to many of my clinical colleagues in Newcastle upon Tyne without whom I would have been unable to offer my patients the wide and comprehensive range of services that are so important in an active oral precancer treatment programme. Of especial importance are those colleagues working in the Departments of Anaesthesia, Medical Physics, Pathology and Medical Photography. Out of these many people, Dr Remani Wariyar in Anaesthetics and Mr Steven Burnett from Medical Physics deserve special mention for their day to day support in the operating theatre.

A manuscript such as this, of course, requires help and cooperation from very many colleagues but, nonetheless, any errors or omissions remain my sole responsibility.

1 Introduction

Peter Thomson

General introduction

This book deals with the diagnosis and management of oral precancer, a relatively rare but important and fascinating range of potentially malignant disorders. Oral precancer comprises both discrete, readily identifiable, oral mucosal lesions such as leukoplakia or erythroplakia and also more widespread or systemic conditions that may affect the lining of the oral cavity, and whose clinical presence may precede the development of invasive oral cancer.

The concept of a recognisable precancer state has arisen following a number of salient clinicopathological observations that include the observed transformation of pre-existing clinical lesions into invasive cancers during patient follow up, the recognition that leukoplakic or erythroplakic lesions are often found to coexist with oral squamous cell carcinoma, and the realisation that numerous histopathological and biomolecular tissue changes are actually common to both cancers and their potentially malignant counterparts [1].

The identification of a potentially malignant disorder in an individual patient, however, does not mean that an inevitable malignant transformation will take place because many of these oral lesions do not progress over time and some may even resolve or regress spontaneously. Nonetheless, statistically, such patients are known to remain at an increased risk of developing mouth cancer.

Cancer of the mouth, which is primarily a squamous cell carcinoma arising from the oral mucosa lining, is the sixth most common cancer worldwide and is traditionally seen most frequently in older people [2]. It is a lethal and deforming disease due not only to local tumour invasion, oro-facial tissue destruction and cervical lymph node metastasis, but also because of widespread blood-borne tumour dissemination affecting particularly the lungs and the liver. Worldwide, 5-year survival rates for oral cancers are around 50%, with prognosis worsening with advanced disease and late presentation [2].

Figure 1.1 shows a typical clinical presentation of a large, invasive, squamous cell carcinoma arising posteriorly in the retromolar and palatoglossal regions of the oral cavity (Figure 1.1A), together with an accompanying computed tomography (CT) scan demonstrating extensive tumour spread to the draining cervical lymph nodes (Figure 1.1B). As is often the case, the patient presented late on in the progress of the cancer disease, having been relatively asymptomatic for many months. Of interest in this case are the surrounding mucosal precancer changes of leukoplakia (clearly visible in Figure 1.1A) that may well have preceded the malignancy.

So, despite real advances in diagnosis and management, nearly half of all patients diagnosed with an oral malignancy will die as a direct consequence of their disease. Whilst the number of patients suffering uncontrolled cancer disease at primary sites in the head and neck has reduced in recent years due to improvements in modern treatment protocols, up to a quarter of patients may then go on to develop multiple cancers in the upper aerodigestive tract either synchronously (at the same time) or metachronously (separated by time).

The presentation of multiple lesions in an individual patient is an illustration of widespread epithelial cell instability, which is a hallmark of head and neck squamous carcinoma, and is classically referred to as 'field change' cancerisation. This was the term first proposed by Slaughter in 1953, who proposed that oral cancers developed in multifocal areas of precancer change as a result of widespread abnormalities in the aerodigestive tract epithelium [3]. More recent observations suggest that the risk of multiple primary cancer development is probably highest in younger patients and particularly in those who continue to smoke and consume alcohol following treatment interventions [2].

(A)

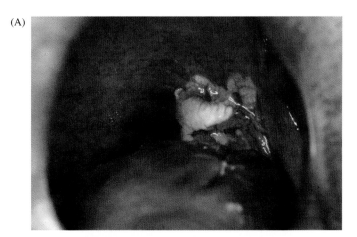

(B)

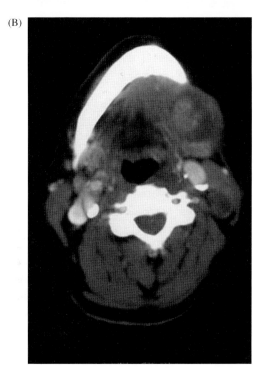

Figure 1.1 (A) Late presenting invasive squamous cell carcinoma (SCC) arising in the retromolar/palatoglossal region. There is surrounding palatal mucosal leukoplakia, precancerous mucosal disease, which probably preceded the malignancy. (B) CT scan illustrating extensive necrotic cervical lymph node tumour spread from retromolar SCC.

Aetiological factors causing malignant transformation of oral stratified squamous epithelium most commonly involve the excessive consumption of tobacco products and alcohol misuse, ultimately presenting clinically as symptomatic tumours in a predominantly elderly male population. In recent years, however, there has been a definite rise in the incidence of oral cancer with higher rates appearing in younger and in female patients. Indeed, no other cancer site has shown such a rapid rise in incidence over the last 25 years and some researchers predict an epidemic of oral cancer occurring during the first half of the 21st century.

Of course, many people who smoke and drink do not develop oral cancer and similarly in a number of other studies it has also been observed that many oral cancer patients may not have been overexposed to tobacco or alcohol at all, so it remains imperative to identify and determine the significance of other potential risk factors. Genetic predisposition to DNA mutation in oral epithelial cells, poor nutrition characterised by a low intake of fresh fruit and vegetables, ageing, low socioeconomic status, poor oral health and infection have all now been implicated in oral carcinogenesis [4].

More recently, a significant role for human papillomavirus (HPV) infection (especially subtype 16) has been postulated in oral carcinogenesis, although this seems to be particularly associated with a rise in oropharyngeal, tonsil and tongue base cancer. This seems to affect young patients in particular, often presenting with extensive cervical lymph node metastases and may be associated with a sexually transmitted aetiology. HPV-associated head and neck cancer may thus represent a distinct disease entity of its own [5,6].

Although HPV DNA has been identified in samples of leukoplakia, the precise role of HPV in the initiation and progression of oral potentially malignant disease remains somewhat obscure and is currently the subject of a number of ongoing investigations.

The 'progression model' for oral carcinogenesis suggests that, following genetic mutation, various phenotypic epithelial tissue disorganisation and dysmaturation changes occur, which if allowed to progress ultimately lead to carcinoma development and invasive disease. Such disorganised features preceding cancer are identifiable at the microscopic level and are described collectively as epithelial dysplasia.

Dysplasia is thus a crucially important histopathological entity that delineates the many structural changes that affect both individual epithelial cells and also the overall integrity of epithelial tissue hierarchy present in potentially malignant lesions. An estimate of the degree of dysplastic change present in the epithelium is made following lesion biopsy and is classified into mild, moderate or severe categories. The more severe the dysplasia, the higher the risk there is for malignant change, although there is a strong subjective element in dysplasia grading and both biopsy sampling errors and possible fluctuations in severity with time may all confound the accuracy of diagnosis.

It has been recognised for many years that a spectrum of distinct oral mucosal abnormalities which may accompany these dysplastic changes can be identified clinically and characterised, albeit somewhat non-specifically, during an oral examination. Figure 1.2 illustrates both the clinical appearance of a diffuse, non-homogenous leukoplakic lesion arising on the ventrolateral tongue mucosa (Figure 1.2A), and its corresponding dysplastic appearance under the microscope (Figure 1.2B).

Fortunately, with the application of a good light source, the oral cavity is easily visualised directly during clinical examination and, indeed, is inspected regularly by dental practitioners during routine dental care. There is, thus, potential for both early diagnosis and therapeutic intervention during this clinically identifiable 'oral precancer window'.

In order to improve survival rates for oral cancer we must therefore avail ourselves of this 'window' to identify precancer change at the earliest possible stage and attempt to intervene to halt the disease process. Unfortunately, there is considerable public ignorance regarding oral cancer, the patient population that is probably most at risk rarely attends for regular oral examination, and general population screening programmes for oral cancer have been found to be fundamentally flawed as a health care intervention.

On the other hand, the identification and targeting of individuals at high risk of developing cancer may provide a more practical solution. For example, it has been shown that many irregular patient attendees who only ever visit dental access centres for emergency treatments are often those with the lifestyle habits that render them most vulnerable to oral cancer. Thus focused oral cancer

(A)

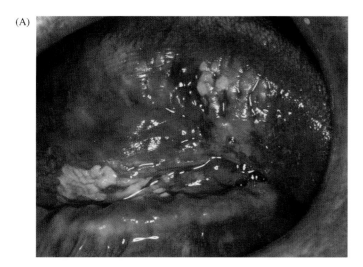

(B)

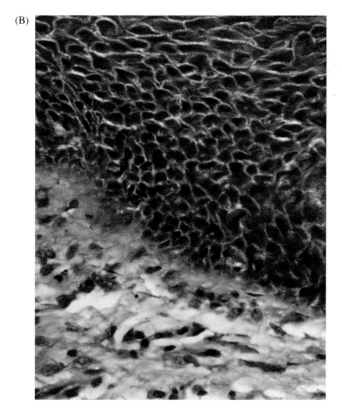

Figure 1.2 (A) Clinical appearance of non-homogenous leukoplakia arising on the ventrolateral tongue mucosa. (B) Accompanying microscopic appearance of the dysplastic tongue epithelium.

screening and health care information may be most effectively targeted to this type of at-risk population group [7].

The currently available scientific literature is also unable to resolve the fundamental question as to whether early diagnosis and treatment of precancerous conditions will ultimately prevent the development of malignant disease. It is not, however, an unreasonable hypothesis and provides a proactive interventional technique that will be discussed in some detail later in this book.

A further problem to consider is that, having identified potentially malignant disorders, we are unable to predict the clinical behaviour of any individual patient or precancer lesion. This common clinical dilemma and its unfortunate consequences are illustrated in Figure 1.3.

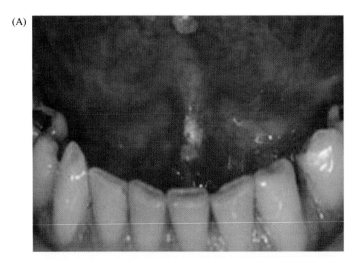

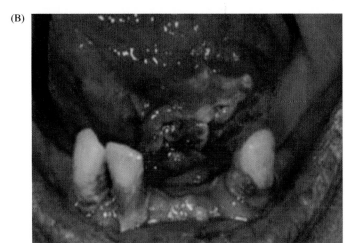

Figure 1.3 (A) Multifocal leukoplakia arising in the anterior floor of the mouth mucosa. How can we predict whether this precancer lesion will progress? (B) In a different patient, an established squamous cell carcinoma presents in the anterior floor of the mouth. How do we know whether this tumour was preceded by a clinically detectable precursor lesion?

There are also no clear management guidelines or agreed treatment strategies for oral precancer cases. The lack of meaningful, randomised controlled clinical trials has resulted in a variety of proposed treatments that are essentially based on clinicians' preferences and experience.

In order to try to address some of these longstanding dilemmas, this book will attempt to concisely review current concepts of oral precancer disease, epithelial cell biology and oral carcinogenesis and its related pathology to try to improve our understanding of this complex and fascinating oral oncology pathway. Utilising a number of longitudinal patient cohort studies, we will also outline our preferred diagnosis and management strategy for potentially malignant disorders and explain our rationale for clinical decision making and treatment selection. It is hoped that in this way we can make a significant contribution to the ongoing scientific debate surrounding oral precancer disease and also help to improve the clinical care and outlook for our many patients that present with these important, potentially malignant and life-threatening oral conditions.

Epidemiology

Studies on the causation, distribution and control of disease form the backbone of epidemiological research. The majority of studies that relate to oral carcinogenesis, however, have tended to focus upon oral cancer rather than potentially malignant disease. However, it is not unreasonable to suppose that the disease process remains consistent for both the development of oral precancer and then its subsequent transformation to invasive carcinoma.

Oral squamous cell carcinoma does, of course, pose a major public health problem worldwide, with an annual estimated incidence of around 275 000 cases of intra-oral cancer. There is a marked variation in global incidence that probably corresponds to varying risk factor behaviours, especially those relating to tobacco smoking or betel-chewing habits and excessive alcohol consumption [2].

The highest rates of oral cancer are seen in Southeast Asia, tropical South America and in parts of Central and Eastern Europe, particularly northern France and Hungary [8]. In the UK there are approximately 5000 new cases of oral cancer seen each year, which actually exceeds the numbers of new cervical cancer, ovarian cancer or leukaemia cases [2]. Even within the UK there are significant regional variations in disease presentation, with Scotland and northern England particularly affected by high levels of oral cancer.

In most countries oral cancer tends to be seen more commonly in men and increases in frequency both with advancing age and with low socioeconomic status, although more recent studies in the European Union and the United States suggest that the disease is increasingly presenting in young professional adults and especially in females [2]. As previously discussed, however, this latter observation may apply more to HPV-related head and neck disease.

It is recognised that cancers may arise from longstanding potentially malignant disorders but whether this is true for all oral cancers is unknown and, as a general observation, potentially malignant disorders affecting the oral cavity are considered to be relatively rare. As there are very few meaningful studies in the literature, it remains difficult to be precise regarding accurate estimates of the true incidence of precancer disease, which by definition refers to the number of new oral potentially malignant lesions arising each year.

Prevalence, on the other hand, is the epidemiological measure of how common a disorder is in a specified population at a particular time. A number of such studies have been carried out to characterise the profile of oral precancer disease. Johnson, for example, quotes an overall precancer prevalence figure of 4.2% for a Sri Lankan population [8], whilst Napier and Speight suggest a worldwide prevalence rate of between 1% and 5% for all potentially malignant disorders [9].

Prevalence of oral leukoplakia

Leukoplakia is recognised worldwide as the commonest oral potentially malignant disorder and has therefore received most study. Quoted prevalence figures for intra-oral leukoplakia, however, vary considerably from less than 0.2% to around 27% and also demonstrate distinct differences between countries. Particularly high prevalence figures, for example, are seen in the Indian subcontinent, Taiwan and New Guinea, which are the regions in which tobacco-chewing habits are especially common, whereas much lower estimates of only 1–2% are proposed for Western populations [8,10].

Petti attempted to estimate a global prevalence figure for leukoplakia by reviewing 23 studies from 17 different countries published between 1986 and 2002 and, by applying a variety of epidemiological analyses, calculated pooled estimates of between 1.5% and 2.6% dependent upon methodology [10]. Unfortunately, there are fundamental problems with epidemiological studies such as these. Not only are they usually very expensive and time-consuming to carry out, but it is also difficult to ensure that a truly representative sample of the desired population has been studied. It may also be extremely difficult to ensure that a consistent and reliable diagnostic method is applied to both the recognition and recording of oral lesions and the findings from one population are not necessarily applicable to the wider population at large [10].

Prevalence figures reported for leukoplakic lesions will also vary significantly between hospital/specialist clinic-based studies where much higher levels of disease from a referred patient base are likely to be seen, compared with data obtained from screening a more generalised population in a community-based setting. Such epidemiological studies rarely include any form of histopathological confirmation of their clinical diagnoses, nor do they reliably comment on the presence or absence of dysplasia in individual lesions.

A further complication occurs when attempts are then made to estimate the proportion of oral cancer cases attributable to malignant transformation of leukoplakia. Whilst figures as high as 17–35% have been quoted for the fraction of oral cancers that are likely to arise from pre-existing leukoplakias [10], these percentages vary significantly between different countries and between study populations and provide virtually no help at all in individual patient counselling and prognosis.

Prevalence of oral erythroplakia

Erythroplakia is known to be much rarer than leukoplakia and there are even fewer data available relating to prevalence figures. Johnson, however, does quote rates of between 0.02% and 0.1% in an Indian subcontinent population [8]. Such lack of information is unfortunate because most studies suggest that eryrthroplakic lesions are at a much higher risk of malignant transformation than leukoplakia and may actually be the most common early clinical sign of an invasive carcinoma; they are therefore probably of much more relevance in the study of oral carcinogenesis.

Although detailed information regarding the incidence and prevalence of potentially malignant disorders remains limited, the recognition of the principal aetiological agents, the types of risk factor behaviour and the subpopulations most at risk of disease development is integral to the proper design and effective delivery of clinical management strategies. Central to any interventional management protocol, of course, must be the prevention of disease.

Prevention

The prevention of oral cancer is of fundamental importance in view of the serious morbidity and mortality consequent upon fully established oral malignant disease. There are, of course, a number of classic tiers of preventive medicine, all of which are relevant to our discussions on the diagnosis and management of oral potentially malignant disorders.

The aim of *primary* prevention is to entirely avoid the development of disease. It thus concentrates on eliminating the principal risk factors of disease and promoting protective behaviour within a community or population. For oral cancer, this clearly includes limiting the use of tobacco, discouraging chewing habits, avoiding excessive alcohol consumption and improving diet. Whilst this seems an eminently sensible approach, especially for patients presenting with precancer lesions, we shall see just how difficult it can be in practice to influence individual patient risk factor behaviour.

Secondary prevention refers to the detection of premalignant or early malignant disease at a stage at which intervention may lead either to an outright cure or to a significant reduction in morbidity and mortality. This approach is highly pertinent to the management of oral potentially malignant disease and will be discussed in detail later in this book.

Finally, the role of *tertiary* prevention is to ultimately reduce the risk of disease recurrence following the treatment of an established condition and to then minimise the risk of disease-related complications. This also has an important place in the overall management strategy for oral precancer patients and is especially relevant during long-term patient follow up after treatment.

We will see in subsequent chapters of this book exactly how, in the context of both the initial diagnosis and then the interventional management of oral potentially malignant disorders, each of these preventive techniques have an important part to play.

Treatment strategies

For the fully established oral squamous cell carcinoma, treatment usually requires surgical ablation of the primary tumour together with a neck dissection to eliminate cervical lymph node metastases, often combined with adjuvant postoperative radiotherapy to the head and neck. HPV-positive disease, on the other hand, often appears to respond particularly well to chemoradiotherapy treatment modalities alone [6].

It is evident, however, that the application of such aggressive treatment modalities can result in significant morbidity to patients, especially in relation to form and function of the mouth and face. Any therapeutic approach that can thus intervene to diagnose oral cancer at a premalignant phase or even at an early invasive stage and institute curative treatment is to be embraced and encouraged.

Oral potentially malignant disorders are, by definition, mucosal conditions only and thus do not require treatments that damage the integrity of important underlying oro-facial structures. This is clearly a significant advantage when compared to the extensive disruption resulting from anti-cancer therapies. In Chapter 8 of this book we will discuss in some detail the treatment methods that have been applied to try to treat oral premalignant lesions and we will outline our preferred interventional management strategy.

Terminology

The natural history of potentially malignant disorders is, unfortunately, not only highly inconsistent but also unpredictable. Both the terminology applied and the definitions used to describe clinical conditions vary considerably in the oral precancer literature, often compounded by confusion between clinical and histological diagnosis. Review and clarification of the terms used in this book are important at the outset and thus the following definitions are formalised here for the reader:

- *Oral cancer (or mouth cancer)*, which strictly includes any malignant neoplasm arising within the oral cavity, is the term used primarily to describe squamous cell carcinoma arising from the oral mucosal lining (OSCC).

- *Oral carcinogenesis* is the multistep process, derived from an accumulation of cellular changes induced by carcinogens, that transforms normal epithelium into invasive neoplasms.

- *Oral precancer* is an overall term describing a range of potentially malignant disorders, both discrete oral mucosal lesions and more generalised conditions, that affect the lining of the oral cavity, imply underlying epithelial tissue disorganisation and dysmaturation, and whose clinical presence may precede the development of oral cancer.

- *Oral precancerous or premalignant lesions*: Traditionally, this 1978 World Health Organisation (WHO) term describes discrete areas of morphologically altered tissue in which there is an increased incidence of cancer compared with apparently normal-looking mucosa. These lesions comprise leukoplakia, erythroplakia and erytholeukoplakia (or speckled leukoplakia).

- *Leukoplakia* is thus a clinical term describing a white patch on the oral mucosa that cannot be wiped off (distinguishing it from pseudomembranous candidosis), and that cannot be characterised clinically or histopathologically as any other definable lesion. Such diagnosis by 'exclusion' implies an underlying epithelial disorder and an increased, but unquantifiable, risk of cancer development.

- *Erythroplakia*, similarly, is defined as a fiery red patch on the oral mucosa that cannot be characterised clinically or pathologically as any other definable disease and which has an enhanced potential for malignant transformation and cancer development. (The older term erythroplasia is rarely used nowadays.)

- *Erythroleukoplakia* (or speckled leukoplakia) is the term given to mixed red and white mucosal patches which display an increased risk of cancer development.

- *Oral precancerous or premalignant conditions*: This 1978 WHO term describes more generalised states in which there is an increased risk of cancer development. It includes a variety of medical disorders such as immunosuppression, iron deficiency anaemia, dermatological disease and chronic infection.

- *Potentially malignant disorders (PMDs)*: This is now the preferred 2005 WHO term, replacing the terms 'precancerous' or 'premalignant' to emphasise a 'potential' (but by no means certain) risk of malignant transformation. It abandons the distinction between discrete lesions and more generalised conditions.

- *Dysplasia* is a histopathological diagnosis that describes a varying presence of epithelial tissue disorganisation, dysmaturation and disturbed cell proliferation. Graded by extent into mild, moderate or severe categories, the most disordered tissue is felt to display the highest risk of malignant transformation.

- *Oral epithelial dysplasia (OED)* is a diagnostic term often applied in the published literature to describe the above histopathological changes seen in oral potentially malignant disorders.

- *Oral precursor lesion* is a relatively non-specific clinical term given to any identifiable pre-existing lesion in which subsequent malignant transformation occurs. Such lesions do not always fall into recognisable potentially malignant categories, nor do they necessarily exhibit dysplasia.

- *Malignant transformation* is the term used to describe same-site transformation of a previously identified precancer into an invasive squamous cell carcinoma.

- *Oral squamous cell carcinoma development* is a term used when patients with pre-existing or previously treated precancer lesions develop invasive carcinoma at new oral sites, distinct from their original lesions.

- *Persistent disease* describes precancer lesions that persist at the same site following treatment.

- *Recurrent disease* describes precancer lesions that reappear at the same site following treatment which had apparently brought about clinical resolution.

- *Further disease* is the term used to describe the development of additional precancer lesions at new, distinct sites in the oral cavity, sometimes appearing after successful treatment of pre-existing lesions.

- *Clinical resolution* refers to the successful removal or regression of a previously identifiable precancer lesion resulting in clinically normal-looking oral mucosa.

- *Field change cancerisation* is the term used to describe a widespread precancer change in any area of mucous membrane exposed to potential carcinogens, thus rendering patients susceptible to multiple lesion disease.

- *Single lesion disease* describes the disease occurring in patients in whom a precancer lesion (of variable size and shape) arises in one, distinct anatomical site.

- *Multiple lesion disease* is defined by the appearance of one or more (sometimes many) precancer lesions, separated by clinically normal-looking areas of oral mucosa.

Summary

The term potentially malignant disorder has now become the recommended nomenclature for oral precancer, not only because it emphasises that not all clinical conditions included under this heading will inevitably transform into cancer but because it also recognises the widespread, often multifocal nature of such disease within the upper aerodigestive tract. Estimates of the prevalence of oral potentially malignant disorders suggest an overall figure of between 2%

and 3%, with the vast majority of lesions associated with tobacco use, appearing clinically as leukoplakias and usually presenting in older, male patients. A uniform use of clinicopathological terminology is recommended not only when managing patients, but also when undertaking teaching and research. An accurate prediction of which patients or indeed which potentially malignant lesions may progress to carcinoma, however, remains elusive so that all precancer patients must be regarded as being at high risk of malignant transformation.

References

1. Warnakulasuriya S, Johnson NW, van der Waal I. Nomenclature and classification of potentially malignant disorders of the oral mucosa. *J Oral Pathol Med* 2007, 36: 575–580.
2. Warnakulasuriya S. Global epidemiology of oral and oropharyngeal cancer. *Oral Oncol* 2009; 45: 309–316.
3. Slaughter DP, Southwick HW, Smejkal W. Field cancerization in oral stratified squamous epithelium: clinical implications of multicentric origin. *Cancer* 1953; 6: 963–968.
4. Warnakulasuriya S. Causes of oral cancer – an appraisal of controversies. *Br Dent J* 2010; 207: 471–475.
5. Mehanna H, Paleri V, West CML, Nutting C. Head and neck cancer.Part 1: Epidemiology, presentation, and prevention. *Br Med J* 2010; 341: 663–666.
6. Mehanna H, West CML, Nutting C, Paleri V. Head and neck cancer. Part 2: Treatment and prognostic factors. *Br Med J* 2010; 341: 721–725.
7. Williams M, Bethea J. Patient awareness of oral cancer health advice in a dental access centre: a mixed methods study. *Br Dent J* 2011; 210: E9.
8. Johnson NW. *Global epidemiology*. In: Shah JP, Johnson NW, Batsakis JG (eds) *Oral Cancer*. London: Martin Dunitz, 2003: 3–32.
9. Napier SS, Speight PM. Natural history of potentially malignant oral lesions and conditions: an overview of the literature. *J Oral Pathol Med* 2008; 37: 1–10.
10. Petti S. Pooled estimate of world leukoplakia prevalence: a systematic review. *Oral Oncol* 2003; 39: 770–780.

2 Form and Function of the Oral Mucosa

C. Max Robinson and Peter Thomson

Oral Precancer: Diagnosis and Management of Potentially Malignant Disorders, First Edition. Edited by Peter Thomson.
© 2012 John Wiley & Sons, Ltd. Published 2012 by John Wiley & Sons, Ltd.

Introduction

The oral cavity is lined by a stratified squamous epithelium which, together with its underlying lamina propria of fibrovascular connective tissue, has a structure and function that varies from site to site in the oral cavity. It is hardly surprising, therefore, that the incidence of oral mucous membrane disease is influenced by both anatomical structure and physiological function.

In Northern European patients, intraoral squamous cell carcinoma predominates in the ventrolateral tongue, floor of mouth and mandibular alveolus regions. These areas have been postulated to form a 'gutter zone' into which soluble carcinogens may pool and exert their neoplastic influence. Figure 2.1 illustrates an invasive squamous cell carcinoma arising from the floor of mouth tissue. In contrast, squamous cancers are rare on the tongue dorsum and hard palate.

There are probably underlying structural and functional distinctions that contribute to the increased risk of oral carcinogenesis at certain oral sites. It is thus important to have a clear understanding of both the applied anatomy of the oral cavity and the cellular biology of its lining oral mucous membrane.

Applied anatomy of the oral cavity

The border between the facial skin and the vermilion of the lip, the mucocutaneous junction, defines the entry to the oral cavity. The vermillion of the lip is continuous with the labial mucosa, which becomes the buccal mucosa beyond the commissure or corners of the mouth and extends backwards until it attaches to the alveolar ridges and pterygomandibular raphe. Whilst potentially malignant lesions may present not infrequently at labial commissure regions, as shown in Figure 2.2, invasive cancers affecting the buccal mucosa tend in general to arise more posteriorly.

The posterior limits of the oral cavity are defined by the palatoglossal folds, the junction of the hard and soft palate and the line of circumvallated papillae that separates the anterior two-thirds of the tongue (oral or mobile part of the tongue) from the posterior third of the tongue (base of tongue). The anterior two-thirds of the tongue extends from the circumvallated papillae forward to its undersurface, where it then attaches to the floor of the mouth. The mobile

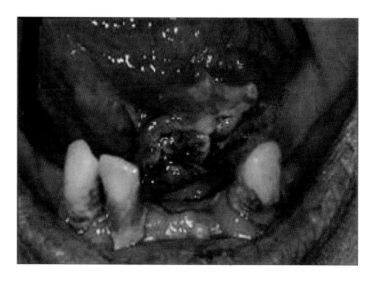

Figure 2.1 Squamous cell carcinoma arising from floor of mouth tissue.

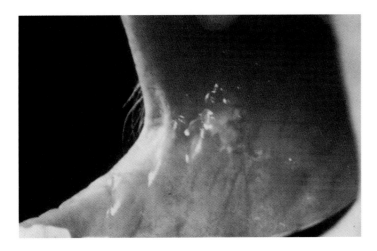

Figure 2.2 Labial commissure leukoplakia extending to the buccal mucosa.

tongue comprises a tip, lateral borders and both dorsal and ventral surfaces. Disease incidence varies considerably between tongue sites, with the dorsum and tongue tip rarely affected by squamous cell carcinoma, whilst the ventro-lateral tongue is a particularly common site for both malignant and premalignant disease (Figure 2.3).

The superior part of the oral cavity is formed anteriorly by the hard palate, which separates the oral cavity from the nose, and more posteriorly by the mobile soft palate, which extends backwards into the oropharynx.

The inferior oral cavity is defined by the floor of the mouth, which is in continuity with the ventral surface of the oral tongue. Whilst the tongue occupies most of the floor, the sublingual region describes the tissues underneath the tongue tip and sides, and contains the submandibular salivary gland ducts which open anteriorly. The sublingual region is divided into left and right by the midline lingual fraenum. The vast majority of floor of mouth cancers and potentially malignant lesions arise anteriorly, as illustrated in Figures 2.1 and 2.4, respectively.

More posteriorly sited within the floor of the mouth are the sublingual salivary gland and lingual nerve, which lie in the immediate submucosal tissues. Whilst fewer malignant lesions arise in the posterior floor of the mouth, these structures are often compromised either by local disease extension or during surgical lesion excision.

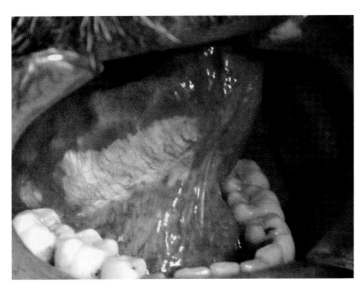

Figure 2.3 Leukoplakia presenting on the ventrolateral tongue. Note the extension of the lesion posterolaterally along the tongue surface.

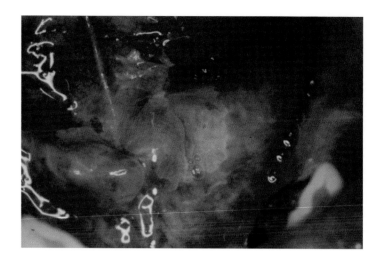

Figure 2.4 Anterior floor of the mouth showing the opening of the submandibular ducts. In this patient there is feint, homogeneous leukoplakia overlying the ducts and spreading towards the lingual mucosa.

The alveolar process that bears the teeth is invested by alveolar mucosa that makes the transition to the gingiva, which forms a cuff around the necks of the teeth. Although the upper and lower alveolar ridges are anatomically distinct, both the structure and function of this mucosa and the incidence of disease are identical at both sites. Figure 2.5 shows an extensive erythroleukoplakic lesion arising from the posterior mandibular alveolus which has already transformed into an invasive carcinoma.

Immediately posterior to the oral cavity is the oropharynx, which comprises the palatine tonsils, the base of the tongue and the soft palate. The soft palate, the anterior and posterior faucial pillars (which surround the palatine tonsils) and the retromolar trigone (a triangular mucosal region covering the ascending ramus of mandible) together form a high-risk site for oral cancer development (Figure 2.6) [1–3].

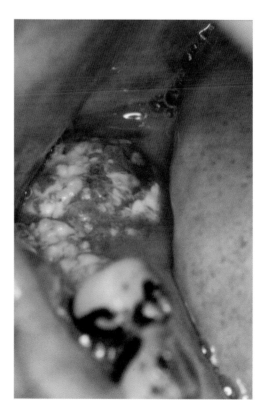

Figure 2.5 Erythroleukoplakia arising in the mandibular alveolar mucosa. This lesion has progressed to become an invasive squamous cell carcinoma.

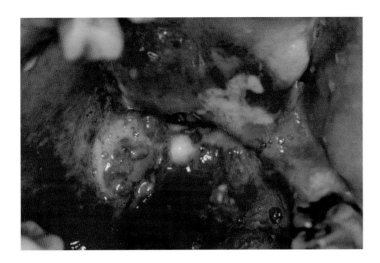

Figure 2.6 Extensive, destructive squamous cell carcinoma arising in the soft palate and extending into the oropharynx.

Function of the oral mucosa

The oral mucosa lines the oral cavity and is covered by a thin film of saliva. It comprises a surface squamous epithelium with an underlying lamina propria. When the mucosa lies directly on bone it is termed mucoperiosteum, but elsewhere there is a submucosa which is composed of parenchymal fibro-adipose tissue and contains lobules of minor salivary glands and neurovascular bundles. Below the submucosa are the deep anatomical structures of the oro-facial complex, including the muscles of mastication, the major salivary glands and the maxillae.

The oral cavity is a complex environment that is adapted for the mastication and ingestion of food, taste sensation, speech and extrinsic antigen surveillance. The oral mucosa forms a physical barrier that protects the submucosal structures from the mechanical, thermal and chemical challenges associated with the consumption of food. It is also an important sensory organ that detects touch, proprioception, temperature, pain and taste sensations. The oral mucosa, along with saliva and the normal oral flora, provides protection against infection from pathogenic microorganisms. It is also an important portal for antigen sampling, priming the immune system for an appropriate and rapid response.

Microanatomy of the oral mucosa

The squamous epithelium is composed of keratinocytes that are organised into a multilayered, stratified structure. The epithelium has a basal cell layer, prickle cell layer, granular cell layer and keratinised or cornified layer. The basal keratinocytes are attached to the basement membrane; the epithelial–mesenchymal interface, which is continuous with the lamina propria. The basal cells are attached to the basement membrane by specialised structures called hemi-desmosomes. Desmosomes are the strong intercellular contacts between keratinocytes that preserve the integrity of the entire epithelium.

The basal cells proliferate and produce new cells that maintain the thickness of the epithelium as cells are lost by desquamation at the surface. The basal cells include stem cells and transit-amplifying cells that are organised into units. The stem cell divides to produce another stem cell and a transit-amplifying cell. The transit-amplifying cell then undergoes several rounds of mitosis, producing the large numbers of daughter cells required to populate the epithelium.

The stem cell divides infrequently, but the transit-amplifying cells have a shorter cell cycle and divide more frequently. Cell cycle kinetics maintain the oral epithelium in equilibrium and enable epithelial regeneration following injury. The turnover time for oral epithelium is longer than that of gastrointestinal epithelium (4–14 days), but shorter than that for the epidermis (52–75 days). The turnover time for buccal epithelium is around 25 days and for gingiva 50 days [3].

Following rounds of cell division, the transit-amplifying cells commit to terminal differentiation. The cells loose the capacity to divide and start to accumulate cytoplasmic intermediate filaments called cytokeratins (CKs). There are numerous CK molecules that are classified into two groups: basic high molecular weight and acidic low molecular weight CKs. The CKs form pairs and have distinct spatial expression within the epithelial layers; CK5 and CK14 are expressed in the basal cells, CK4 and CK13 are expressed in non-keratinised squamous epithelium, and CK1 and CK10 are expressed by keratinised epithelium [4].

These differentiating cells form the prickle cell layer, which refers to the appearance of the 'spiky' profile of the keratinocytes in formalin-fixed, paraffin-embedded tissue sections stained with haematoxylin and eosin (H&E). The spikes or spines represent the desmosomal intercellular attachments. In addition to cytokeratins, several other structural proteins accumulate, for example loricrin, filaggrin and involucrin [4].

In non-keratinised squamous epithelium the surface layers are composed of polygonal keratinocytes. By contrast, in parakeratinised epithelium the keratinocytes become flattened and the nucleus becomes pyknotic (shrunken) and hyperchromatic (darker). Terminally differentiated squamous cells are eventually lost by desquamation at the surface. Orthokeratinisation is characterised by a granular cell layer between the prickle cell layer and the surface squames. The granular cell layer is replete with coarse keratohyaline bodies, which produce the typical granular appearance in H&E-stained tissue sections. The surface squamous cells, just a few cells thick, do not contain any discernable nuclear material and are termed anucleate squames.

Whilst most of the epithelium is composed of keratinocytes, there are also melanocytes (around one per ten basal keratinocytes), scattered Langerhans' cells and neurosensory cells, Merkel cells and taste bud structures. Melanocytes produce melanin in varying amounts, accounting for racial pigmentation within the oral cavity, whilst Langerhans' cells are antigen-presenting cells and form part of the mucosal immune defence system [5].

The lamina propria is the connective tissue or mesenchyme that lies immediately below the epithelium. It is divided into the superficial papillary layer and the deeper reticular layer. The papillary lamina propria interdigitates with the rete processes of the epithelium. The lamina propria is composed of fibrous tissue that is ramified by a rich neurovascular supply. The fibrous tissue contains fibroblasts, myofibroblasts and fibrocytes that elaborate collagen and elastin fibres along with other glycoproteins and proteoglycans that form the ground substance of the lamina propria [5].

Collagen is the most abundant constituent of the lamina propria, forming around 60% of the overall structure, and imparts mechanical strength. Together with the other proteins, a structure is produced which is well adapted for the compression and stretching that occurs during mastication, swallowing and speech. The lamina propria also contains transiting immune Langerhans' cells, macrophages, mast cells and B and T lymphocytes which, together with the epithelial component, completes the mucosal immune defence system.

Interactions between the epithelium and the lamina propria are essential for homeostatic maintenance of the mucosa. Such interactions are essential for epithelial cell proliferation and differentiation, and are also involved in extracellular matrix remodelling. This mucosal maintenance programme is mediated by families of cell adhesion molecules, for example the cadherins (epithelia–epithelial cell adhesion molecules) and the integrins (cell–extracellular matrix adhesion molecules), along with the influence of multiple growth factors (e.g. epidermal growth factor, platelet-derived growth factor, transforming growth factor, keratinocyte growth factor) and cytokines (interleukins) [4].

Deregulation of the complex interactions between epithelium and underlying connective tissue inevitably has a part to play in the development of oral precancer and the pathogenesis of oral squamous cell carcinoma [3].

Regional variation of the oral mucosa

The clinical appearance of the oral mucosa is dependent on the thickness of the epithelium, the amount of surface keratinisation, melanin pigmentation and the vascularity of the lamina propria. There are three prototypic mucosal patterns: lining mucosa, masticatory mucosa and the specialised mucosa that covers the dorsum of the tongue. These mucosal differences are summarised in Table 2.1 [3–5].

Lining mucosa

The vermillion border of the *lip* is covered by a thin, stratified squamous epithelium that shows orthokeratinisation. The lamina propria of the vermillion is highly vascular, producing the characteristic red colour typically seen in Caucasians. This redness is modified by increasing amounts of melanin in other racial groups, which imparts a brown colouration.

By contrast, the *labial mucosa* and *buccal mucosa* are covered by a thick, non-keratinised, stratified squamous epithelium (Figure 2.7A). The prickle cell layer often contains glycogen-rich keratinocytes that produce areas of vacuolated cells. Although the labial and buccal mucosae are mainly covered by non-keratinised squamous epithelium, in reality there is functional adaption in areas such as the occlusal plane where constant mechanical trauma causes light parakeratosis; the resultant clinical appearance of a white line along the occlusal plane is the 'linea alba', and in cheek biting habits this can be quite pronounced (Figure 2.8).

Site	Squamous epithelium	Lamina propria	Clinical appearance
Lining mucosa			
Vermilion of lip	Thin Orthokeratinised	Fibrovascular tissue	Red and fissured
Labial and buccal mucosa	Thick Non-keratinised	Fibrous tissue	Pink and smooth
Floor of mouth, ventrum tongue and alveolar mucosa	Thin Non-keratinised	Fibrovascular tissue	Red and smooth
Masticatory mucosa			
Hard palate and gingival	Thick Para-/orthokeratinised	Dense fibrous tissue	Pink and stippled
Specialised mucosa			
Dorsum of tongue	See text	Fibrovascular tissue	Pink and velvety

Table 2.1 Regional variation of the oral mucosa.

(A)

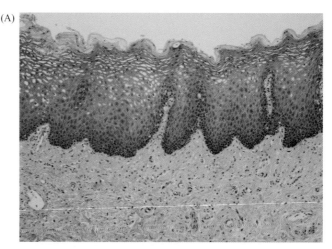

(B)

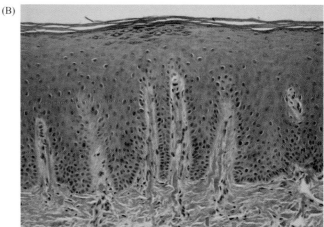

Figure 2.7 Photomicrographs of oral mucosae stained with H&E showing (A) non-keratinised buccal mucosa and (B) keratinised palatal mucosa.

The lamina propria is composed of fibrous tissue that contains an elastin fibre-rich scaffold that facilitates stretch and recoil during mastication, speech and swallowing. The epithelial–mesenchymal interface is characterised by rete processes that are elongated, broad and branching, presumably contributing to the stretchiness of the mucosa. The thickness of the epithelium and fibroelastic lamina propria imparts a light pink colouration to the mucosa.

The *floor of the mouth* and the *ventral tongue* are covered by thin, non-keratinised squamous epithelium. The lamina propria is composed of

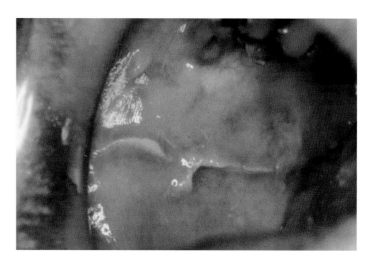

Figure 2.8 Hyperkeratosis on the buccal mucosa along the occlusal line of the teeth ('linea alba'), which in this case is pronounced due to repetitive cheek biting.

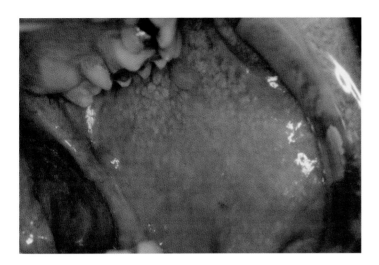

Figure 2.9 Collection of sebaceous glands within the submucosa of the buccal tissue (Fordyce's spots).

fibrovascular tissue. The epithelial–mesenchymal interface is rather flat in profile and the rete processes are fewer and shallower than in buccal and labial mucosae. The combination of a thin epithelium and a vascular lamina propria produces a reddish clinical appearance.

The lining mucosa is perforated by the ducts of the major salivary glands: Wharton's duct, the main collecting duct of the submandibular gland, opens at the submandibular papillae in the anterior floor of the mouth, whilst Stenson's duct, draining the parotid, opens at a prominent papilla on the buccal mucosa opposite the upper first permanent molar tooth. Multiple ducts of Rivinus open into the anterior floor of the mouth from the sublingual gland and there are thousands of minor salivary glands throughout the oral cavity that also empty their contents on to the surface of the mucosa.

Numerous sebaceous glands are located at the mucocutaneous border of the lip, visible by their slight yellowish hue, and are positioned intra-orally near the commissure regions of the buccal mucosa where they are termed Fordyce's spots (Figure 2.9).

Masticatory mucosa

The *hard palate* and *gingivae* are covered by masticatory mucosa, which is adapted to withstand the mechanical forces generated during mastication. The mucosa is firmly bound down to the underlying bone surface to produce a tough mucoperiosteum composed of dense fibrous tissue. The mucosa is covered by a relatively thick squamous epithelium. The palate is mainly covered by ortho-keratinised squamous epithelium and the rete process are numerous, long and spiky (Figure 2.7B).

The gingiva is the mucosal structure that forms an attachment to the emergent teeth. The attached gingiva bound to alveolar bone and the external part of the free gingiva are both covered by parakeratinised and orthokeratinised squamous epithelium. The free gingiva that lies adjacent to the crown of the tooth is lined by sulcular epithelium which is non-keratinised. The latter is adapted for the transudation of gingival crevicular fluid and the emigration of immune cells, mainly neutrophils, in response to bacterial plaque accumulation. In health, the attached and free gingivae are light pink in colour and have a stippled appearance. The attached gingiva forms a scalloped border with the alveolar mucosa, which is redder in colour and covered by a thin, non-keratinised squamous epithelium.

Specialised mucosa

The transition from the ventral surface of the tongue to the dorsum marks the beginning of a unique specialised mucosa that shows adaptations for control of the food bolus during mastication and swallowing and is also involved in taste sensation. The mucosa is organised into microanatomical units called *papillae*.

The most numerous are the filiform papillae. These structures have a fibro-connective tissue core that is covered by stratified squamous epithelium, the surface of which bears slender tiers of parakeratinised squames. The arrangement is classically described as resembling a Christmas tree (Figure 2.10A). The

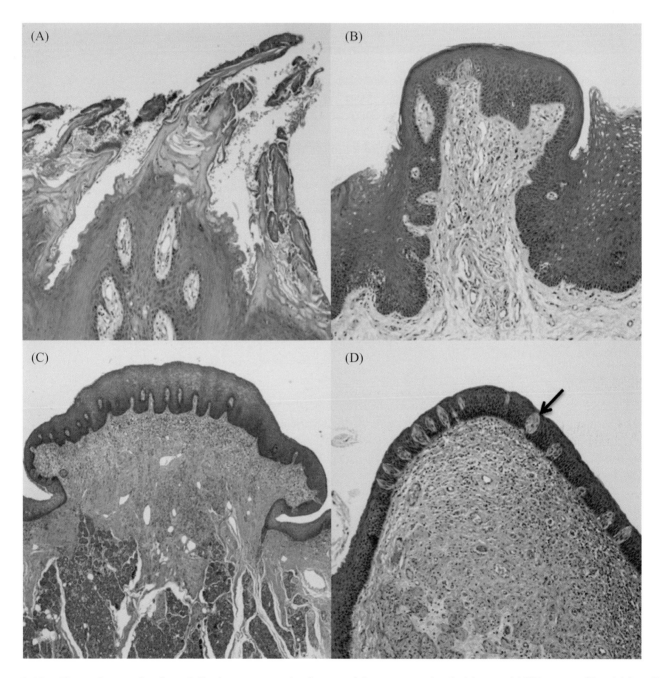

Figure 2.10 Photomicrographs of specialised mucosae on the dorsum of the tongue stained with H&E: (A) filiform papillae, (B) fungiform papilla, (C) circumvalate papilla and (D) foliate papilla showing taste bud structures (arrow) within the epithelium.

filiform papillae give the dorsum of the tongue its characteristic 'furry' or 'velvety' surface.

There are also numerous fungiform papillae, which have a dome-shaped fibroconnective tissue core that is variably covered by non-keratinised and keratinised squamous epithelium (Figure 2.10B). The epithelium incorporates taste bud structures composed of specialised chemoreceptive cells that are innervated by a rich plexus of peripheral nerves.

There are also around 7–15 circumvalate papillae, arrayed in a V-shaped line just anterior to the sulcus terminalis at the junction of the posterior and middle thirds of the tongue. These structures are about 5 mm in diameter and are easily identified during clinical examination. The circumvalate papillae are dome-shaped and have a deep trough around their circumference. They are usually covered by non-keratinised squamous epithelium that incorporates taste buds on the lateral walls of the papilla (Figure 2.10C). At the base of the trough there are serous salivary gland lobules called von Ebner's glands.

The foliate papillae are located on the posterolateral aspect of the oral tongue and are frond-like folds of non-keratinised squamous mucosa that also contain numerous taste bud structures (Figure 2.10D). In addition, the foliate papillae usually have focal areas of mucosal-associated lymphoid tissue, termed lingual tonsil, which has a similar microanatomical structure to pharyngeal tonsil.

Oral epithelial cell kinetics

Oral carcinogenesis is a multistep process resulting in molecular and genetic changes leading to dysregulation of cell proliferation and differentiation, ultimately recognisable as phenotypic changes within the epithelium, and is termed dysplasia. Whilst this will be discussed in more detail in Chapters 3 and 6, it is important to our understanding of the oral mucosal structure to recognise that cells most likely to be associated with premalignant change during carcinogenesis are those with the highest inherent proliferative activity.

As outlined previously, it is within the progenitor compartment of the epithelium, comprising the basal and immediately suprabasal cells, that cell division and renewal takes place. Basal keratinocytes differentiate and migrate through the upper prickle and granular layers to the surface where they are shed as keratin squames. Keratinocytes are thus effectively programmed to divide, differentiate and ultimately die by programmed cell death or apoptosis.

For the maintenance of both the structure and function of the oral mucosa, therefore, cell proliferation, terminal differentiation and spontaneous apoptosis must all remain strictly regulated. Whilst cancer cells presumably evolve an ability to escape from their inherent apoptotic programmes, it is most likely to be within the basal cell progenitor compartment that the first signs of increasing and ultimately dysregulated cell proliferation may be seen [6].

Central to the understanding of cell proliferation is the concept of the cell cycle, which is an ordered set of processes by which one cell grows and divides into two daughter cells. A schematic summary of the cell cycle is illustrated in Figure 2.11. Rapidly dividing epithelial cells have a cycle that lasts around 20 hours, divided into interphase occupying the majority of the cycle and mitosis lasting only about 1 hour. Mitosis is a dramatic, coordinated change in cellular architecture leading to segregation of the chromosomes replicated during the S phase of DNA synthesis prior to the initiation of cell division.

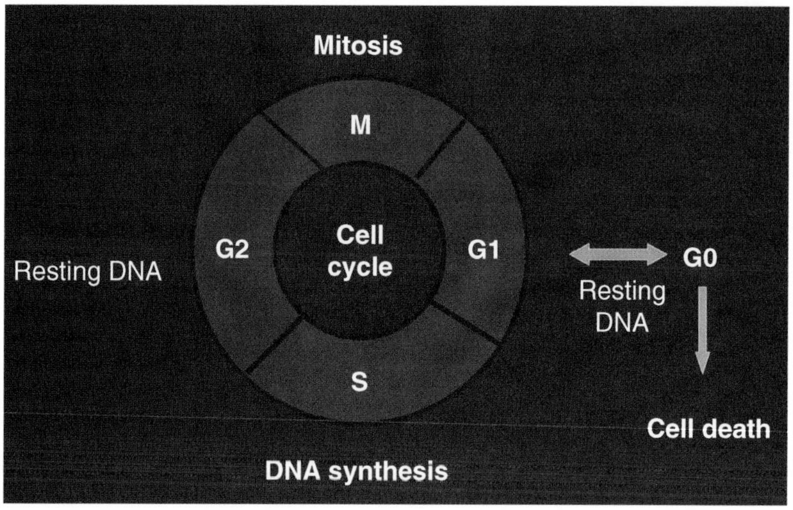

Figure 2.11 Schematic diagram of the cell cycle.

The S phase is preceded by a gap called G1 (postmitotic, presynthetic phase) and followed by a further gap, G2 (postsynthetic, premitotic phase). Following mitosis, and in the absence of cell division stimuli, the majority of cells in normal adult tissue are in a quiescent phase, G0. Following mitogenic stimuli, cells in G0 or G1 progress to a restriction or transition point, after which they are committed to enter the S phase.

The cell cycle and its control is highly complex and, whilst a detailed description is outwith the remit of this book, it is useful to appreciate that while cell progression through cycle phases is facilitated by the synthesis, activation and subsequent degradation of stimulatory cyclin proteins, a variety of inhibitory proteins also act to prevent cell proliferation. Disturbed expression of these regulatory molecules during carcinogenesis, essentially the acquisition of sequential mutations increasing stimulation and decreasing inhibition, leads to loss of cycle control and abnormal proliferative activity [7].

Experimental analysis of the cell cycle and cell proliferation may be performed by labelling newly synthesised DNA with detectable precursor molecules. This was initially achieved using autoradiographic techniques, during which selective uptake of administered radiolabelled thymidine into actively proliferating epithelial cells was measured. However this has now been supplanted by immunohistochemistry and the use of monoclonal antibodies. Antibodies may attach to a variety of proliferation-associated antigens seen during different phases of the cell cycle and are then identified in tissue samples by staining. The great advantage of this latter technique is that it can also be applied to a range of formalin-fixed, paraffin-embedded tissues.

Analytical techniques such as these allow the estimation of labelling indices which effectively calculates the percentage of cells in a tissue sample expressing a particular label, thus enabling a quantitative and reproducible measure of cell proliferative activity to be made. Figure 2.12, for example, illustrates immunohistochemical labelling of cyclin A, a cyclin protein synthesised during the S phase and required both for S phase progression and cell passage from G2 to mitosis in the human floor of mouth mucosa. The interesting feature here is the increased cell proliferation shown by enhanced numbers of labelled cells in epithelial tissue previously diagnosed as dysplastic.

Newer automated techniques such as flow cytometry, based upon dye staining of DNA and subsequent laser excitation and fluorescence analysis, allows thousands of cells to be counted efficiently and provides estimates of the

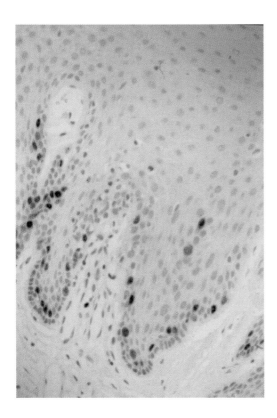

Figure 2.12 Cyclin A-labelled buccal mucosa. Brown staining cells, primarily in the basal and suprabasal layers, represent the progenitor compartment in which DNA synthesis was taking place at the time of labelling.

proportion of cells with varying DNA content. Limitations of this technique exist, however, and include contamination of cell populations with non epithelial inflammatory cells and the lack of tissue structure and hierarchy seen in conventional histological samples. Whilst the latter may be irrelevant in studies of disorganised tumour tissue, it is a major limitation in the investigation of precancer where detailed epithelial structural analysis is integral to the whole diagnostic process.

Oral epithelial cell proliferative activity

Concepts of cell renewal in oral epithelium suggest that epithelial proliferative units exist, possibly represented by the epithelial ridges which are bounded by their connective tissue papillae on either side. Each unit thus effectively shelters the basal cells, amongst which are thought to lie the stem cells, which are those cells with a substantive, synchronous, self-renewal capacity and which are able to constantly renew themselves throughout the lifespan of the individual. Stem cells also, by asymmetrical division, produce daughter keratinocytes which are then irreversibly committed to cellular differentiation [8–10].

As the only cells capable of what is essentially unlimited proliferation, oral keratinocyte stem cells thus play a vitally important role in cell renewal, wound healing and epithelial tissue homeostasis, but they are difficult to identify in tissue samples due to the lack of specific surface markers. This is disappointing from a research point of view because, as the only permanent cells in epithelial tissue capable of unlimited proliferation, stem cells are probably the most likely initial target for carcinogenesis [11,12]. Whilst studies are ongoing to identify and characterise oral keratinocyte stem cells further, particularly in relation to the development of oral squamous carcinoma and its subsequent expansion, invasion and movement through adjacent tissue, oral epithelial proliferation activity can usefully be studied on excised tissue samples as a whole, as outlined above.

'Flash' labelling indices – in which S phase DNA is identified by administering markers of cell proliferative activity to excised tissue in an effort to identify actively dividing cells – remain extremely useful but may, of course, be significantly influenced by the time of day that the tissue is harvested for examination and subsequent labelling. A circadian variation in labelling indices would probably invalidate comparative estimates of cell proliferative activity both within and between individual subjects and also potentially in pathology specimens. Indeed, we have previously observed marked circadian rhythms in proliferation indices in animal cell renewal systems, with peak proliferative activity in mouse tongue epithelium, for example, occurring at 03.00 hours and troughs in activity 12 hours later at 15.00 hours. Figure 2.13 illustrates the histological appearance of labelled cells undergoing DNA synthesis in mouse tongue. A sequential double labelling technique was used whereby an initial radiolabelled thymidine administration (autoradiography) was followed by bromodeoxyuridine (immunohistochemical method). This was used to categorise cell movement to and from the S phase, respectively, together with the total S phase activity calculated from the double cell labelling [8]. Figure 2.14 illustrates a definite cyclical pattern in these labelling indices in mouse tongue, which was recorded by following animals over a 48-hour period.

Most cell proliferation studies have been carried out on animal models and there have been relatively few studies of epithelial cell biology within the human oral mucosa, and those that do exist have tended to primarily

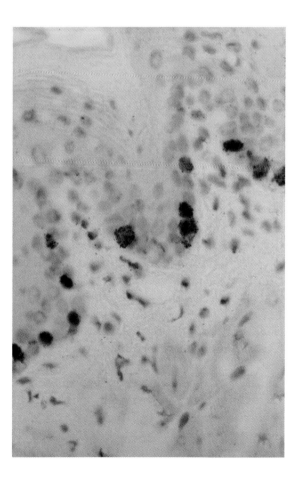

Figure 2.13 Mouse tongue epithelium showing basal cells labelled during the S phase of the cell cycle. In this section, replicating cells have been identified by both autoradiography (silver grains) and immunohistochemistry (brown staining) in a sequential double labelling technique. Subsequent quantitative analysis allows calculation of cell influx to and efflux from the S phase, as well as the overall labelling index.

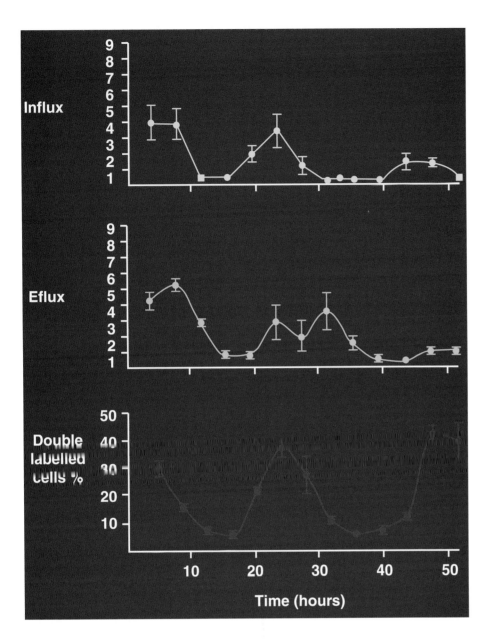

Figure 2.14 Circadian rhythm data for the mouse tongue epithelium based on a double labelling technique which shows movement of cells in and out of the S phase (influx and efflux) and the overall labelling index (total number of cells in S). There are peaks in proliferative activity at 03.00 hours and troughs around 15.00 hours

concentrate on gingival epithelium and its relationship to inflammatory periodontal disease.

As very few data exist on oral cell proliferative activity, we therefore decided to characterise proliferative activity in the human oral cavity by developing an in vitro labelling technique to quantify labelling indices in excised mucosal samples. Initially, taking tissue samples from the buccal mucosa and mandibular gingiva during routine oral surgery procedures, we specifically sought for but found no significant differences between cell proliferative activity observed during the morning hours of 09.00 to 12.00 hours, compared with those examined during the afternoon between 14.00 and 16.00 hours [9]. This important observation suggests that no significant circadian effects influence cell proliferation activity in the human oral mucosa during normal daylight hours, and that a single labelling index obtained during the middle part of the day should be fairly representative of a mean or reference value.

Whilst neither age nor gender appeared to influence oral cell proliferation indices obtained in this study, an important anatomical site distinction was

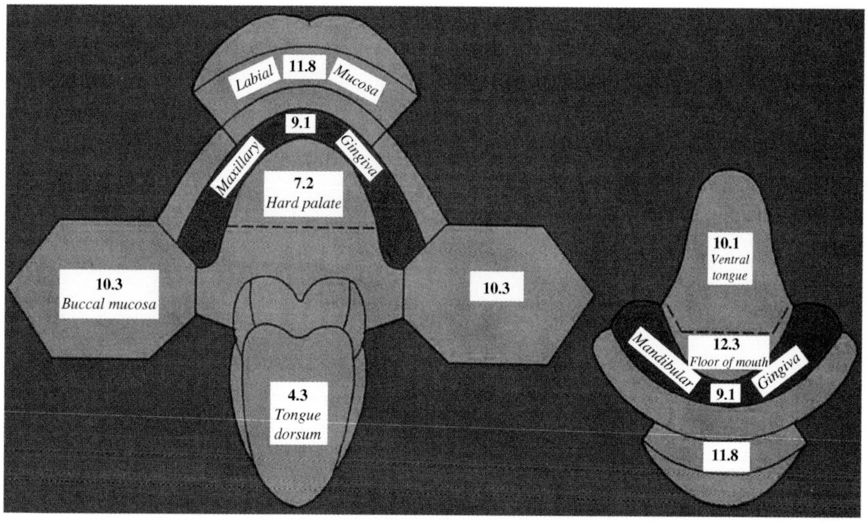

Figure 2.15 Mouth chart summarising cell proliferation labelling indices (%) at eight distinct oral sites: labial and buccal mucosae, maxillary and mandibular gingivae, hard palate, tongue dorsum, ventral tongue and floor of mouth.

observed between non-keratinised lining buccal mucosa, which exhibited a high labelling index of 11.7%, compared with thick, keratinised mandibular gingiva, which showed much lower indices of 8.5% (9).

When this technique was subsequently applied to clinically normal oral tissue harvested from a variety of intra-oral sites (obtained during minor surgical procedures) we were able to construct a cell proliferation profile for the human oral cavity. Subjects were fit and healthy young adults (aged between 20 and 30 years) who were non-smokers and tissue excision was restricted to between 10.00 and 15.00 hours to minimise residual circadian variation [13].

Figure 2.15 summarises on a mouth chart the labelling indices obtained for eight distinct oral sites: labial and buccal mucosae, maxillary and mandibular gingivae, hard palate, tongue dorsum, ventral tongue and floor of mouth. These data confirmed that very high intrinsic proliferative activity was seen in the floor of the mouth (12.3%) and the ventral tongue mucosa (10.1%). Interestingly, not only are these thin, non-keratinised lining mucosae particularly high-risk sites for squamous carcinoma but they are also the regions most prone to mucositis and cytotoxic-induced ulceration during cancer chemotherapy, presumably because of their inherently high proliferative state.

High labelling indices were also seen in the labial (11.8%) and buccal (10.3%) mucosae, which are thicker, non-keratinised mucosae that resemble each other histologically. They provide a lining to the oral cavity, which is often prone to frictional, thermal and chemical irritation. There is, for example, a high incidence of buccal cancers in Southeast Asian populations resulting from long-term tobacco and betel product placement adjacent to the buccal mucosa.

The lowest proliferative labelling activities were seen in the thick, keratinised hard palate mucosa (7.2%) and the specialised tongue dorsum gustatory epithelium (4.3%). These are known to be rare sites for squamous cancer to arise. Both the maxillary and mandibular gingivae were consistent at 9.1%.

Such variation in cell proliferative activity presumably reflects the differing structural and functional demands of the distinct oral mucosal sites, but it is of interest to note how the highest cell proliferation tends to be seen at the sites most frequently affected by precancer or cancer change. It would be of interest to repeat this study in order to compare the young, presumably healthy, oral mucosa profile obtained from this mapping study with a similar mucosal site harvesting exercise from a population of older smoking and drinking patients.

Anatomical site predilection for oral carcinogenesis

Squamous cell carcinoma thus predominates in the floor of the mouth and ventral tongue in Western patient populations. It has often been suggested that the lack of a protective keratin layer and the increased permeability of the thin, lining oral mucosa contributes to rendering these sites more susceptible to the action of soluble carcinogens in tobacco and alcohol [14]. The demonstration of pre-existing, intrinsically high proliferative activity in the floor of the mouth and ventral tongue, however, may represent an important underlying endogenous predisposition to malignant change.

A further and intriguing observation was seen following proliferative labelling of samples of clinically normal-looking floor of mouth and ventral tongue tissue harvested from patients with a previous history of carcinoma. Particularly high mean labelling indices of 14% for the floor of the mouth and 16.2% for the ventral tongue were observed in mucosa taken from these sites, in contrast to their control values of 12.3% and 10.1%, respectively (Figure 2.15). This perhaps once again emphasises the underlying proliferative instability of inherently vulnerable mucosa [15]. As a matter of interest, excised squamous cell carcinomas from these high-risk sites demonstrated even higher mean labelling indices of 15.1% for the floor of the mouth and 15.7% for the ventral tongue, with a trend for increased labelling to be seen in the most poorly differentiated tumours.

It is probable also, therefore, that the similarly observed high cell proliferation rates seen within clinically normal buccal mucosae may contribute, as outlined above, to:

1. The high incidence of buccal tumours in Southeast Asian populations, where tobacco and betel product placement in the buccal sulcus for prolonged periods is commonplace.

2. Lip cancer where the high proliferative activity of labial mucosa may contribute an inherent susceptibility to actinic radiation.

In contrast, the oral sites with the lowest epithelial cell proliferative activity, such as the thick, keratinised or specialised mucosa of the hard palate and tongue dorsum, are relatively rare sites for the development of squamous cancer. Thus, as oral tissue becomes specialised with more complex functional demands, so its capacity for rapid self-renewal becomes limited and proliferative activity decreases. Whilst this may be disadvantageous in terms of rapidity and completeness of tissue repair following injury, it may paradoxically offer a degree of protection against carcinogenesis.

Summary

The structure and function of mucosal lining thus varies from site to site in the oral cavity, as does the frequency of precancer and cancer development. It is unlikely that these observations are coincidental. Increased oral epithelial cell proliferation is seen at sites, particularly the floor of the mouth and ventral tongue, where oral epithelial dysplastic lesions and invasive squamous cell carcinoma are most frequent.

There must also be an important inter-relationship between epithelial tissue and the underlying lamina propria and submucosa. Exactly how these two tissues interact to influence the progression of precancer disease from epithelial dysplasia into invasive carcinoma remains unclear but these mechanisms are undoubtedly of fundamental importance to the process of oral carcinogenesis.

References

1. Slootweg PJ, Eveson JW. Tumours of the oral cavity and oropharynx. In: Barnes L, Eveson J, Reichart P, Sidransky D (eds) *Pathology and Genetics of Head and Neck Tumours (IACR WHO Classification of Tumours)*. Oxford: Oxford University Press, 2005: 166–167.

2. Batsakis JG. Clinical pathology of oral cancer. In: Shah JP, Johnson NW, Batsakis JG (eds) *Oral Cancer*. London: Martin Dunitz, 2003: 75–129.

3. Nanci A. *Ten Cate's Oral Histology: Development, Structure and Function*, 7th edn. St Louis, MO: Mosby Elsevier, 2008: 319–357.

4. Berkovitz BKB, Holland GR, Moxham BJ. *Oral Anatomy, Histology and Embryology*, 4th edn. St Louis, MO: Mosby Elsevier, 2009: 223–252.

5. Sloan P, Picardo M, Schor SL. The structure and function of oral mucosa. *Dent Update* 1991; 18: 208–216.

6. Loro LL, Vintermyr OK, Johannessen AC. Apoptosis in normal and diseased oral tissues. *Oral Dis* 2005; 11: 274–287.

7. Donovan JCH, Slingerland J, Tannock IF. Cell proliferation and tumor growth. In Tannock IF, Hill RP, Bristow RG, Harrington L (eds) *The Basic Science of Oncology*, 4th edn. New York: McGraw-Hill, 2005: 167–193.

8. Thomson PJ, McGurk M, Potten CS, Walton GM, Appleton DR. Tritiated thymidine and bromodeoxyuridine double-labelling studies on growth factors and oral epithelial proliferation in the mouse. *Arch Oral Biol* 1999; 44: 721–734.

9. Thomson PJ, Potten CS, Appleton DR. In vitro labelling studies and the measurement of epithelial cell proliferative activity in the human oral cavity. *Arch Oral Biol* 2001; 46: 1157–1164.

10. Appleton DR, Thomson PJ, Donaghey CE, Potten CS, McGurk M. Simulation of cell proliferation in mouse oral epithelium, and the action of epidermal growth factor: evidence for a high degree of synchronization of the stem cells. *Cell Prolifer* 2002; 35 (Suppl 1): 68–77.

11. Calenic B, Ishkitiev N, Yaegaki K et al. Characterization of oral keratinocyte stem cells and prospects of its differentiation to oral epithelial equivalents. *Romanian J Morphol Embryol* 2010; 51: 641–645.

12. Mackenzie IC. Growth of malignant oral epithelial stem cells after seeding into organotypical cultures of normal mucosa. *J Oral Pathol Med* 2004; 33: 71–78.

13. Thomson PJ, Potten CS, Appleton DR. Mapping dynamic epithelial cell proliferative activity within the oral cavity of man: a new insight into carcinogenesis? *Br J Oral Maxillofac Surg* 1999; 37: 377–383.

14. Mashberg A, Meyers H. Anatomical site and size of 222 early asymptomatic oral squamous cell carcinomas. *Cancer* 1976; 37: 2149–2157.

15. Thomson PJ, Potten CS, Appleton DR. Characterization of epithelial cell activity in patients with oral cancer. *Br J Oral Maxillofac Surg* 1999; 37: 384–390.

3 Oral Carcinogenesis

Peter Thomson

Introduction

It is estimated that approximately one in three people will develop cancer at some point in their life. Cancer affects almost every complex multicellular organism and involves disruption of the processes of cell proliferation, differentiation and development. Understanding cancer is not only important in the fight against malignant disease, but also in helping to improve our understanding of the fundamental biological mechanisms of life itself.

This chapter is concerned with the complex, multistage process of oral carcinogenesis. This is a cumulative sequence of cellular and tissue changes, some of which may be reversible but which if unchecked will ultimately transform normal oral keratinocytes into invasive cancer cells. It is important for us, as clinicians, to understand current pertinent concepts of oral oncology in order to recognise the earliest possible signs of carcinogenesis in our patients and to intervene proactively in the disease process.

Whilst the term oncology literally means the scientific study of new growths, it has become synonymous over the years with the overall study of malignant disease, the mechanisms governing cancer development, its treatment and clinical outcome. Traditionally, a malignant tumour is defined as an abnormal, uncoordinated growth of tissue that persists in an excessive manner after initiating stimuli have ceased and which then progresses to local tissue invasion, destruction and ultimately metastatic spread. In reality, malignant tumours are most likely composed of significantly heterogeneous and dynamic populations of abnormal and mutated cells that undergo constant and rapid cell proliferation and that compete for nutritional resource from both within the tumour and the outside host.

Figure 3.1 shows the histopathological appearance of an oral squamous cell carcinoma, which has arisen from a precursor dysplastic lesion, and which is now invading the underlying connective tissue. The overlying epithelium is no longer intact giving rise to the classic clinical picture of a non-healing, persistent mucosal ulcer.

Cancers may be initiated by various stimuli such as physical, chemical or biological agents and then, often following a latent phase, may be promoted by subsequent non-specific irritation or damage which encourages tumour progression and ultimately metastasis. Box 3.1 summarises these classic stages of initiation, promotion, progression and metastasis, which together form the hallmark of carcinogenesis.

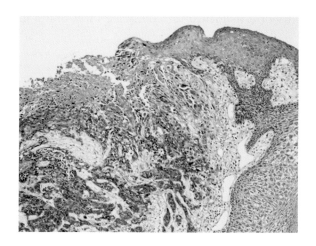

Figure 3.1 Histopathology slide showing an oral squamous cell carcinoma arising from a pre-existing dysplastic lesion. On the surface there is a breach in continuity of the epithelium (ulceration), whilst carcinoma invades the immediately subjacent lamina propria.

Box 3.1 Classic stages in the development of cancer.

- *Initiation*: This is an irreversible process of DNA mutation, probably in stem cells, which follows damage induced by carcinogens. Mutagens may be physical, chemical or biological in nature
- *Promotion*: Following a variable latent phase and, only after initiation, non-specific circumstances selectively 'promote' the expansion of altered cells, but are ineffective in producing cancer on their own. Cycles of initiation and promotion may exist before final emergence of the malignant phenotype
- *Progression*: Increasing tissue disorganisation leads to a preinvasive state before finally progressing to malignant transformation, tissue invasion and local spread of disease
- *Metastasis*: The unequivocal hallmark of malignancy is the detachment and embolisation of tumour deposits, which effectively spreads disease from one body site to another, usually via the bloodstream or lymphatics. Metastases or secondary tumours are thus discontinuous with the primary tumour and are the major cause of death from malignant disease

It is now recognised, of course, that cancer is fundamentally a genetic disorder caused by the accumulation of multiple mutations in cellular DNA and, whilst the concepts of initiation, promotion and progression remain relevant, it is really a disease that is characterised by the complexity of its aetiological mechanisms. It is probable that the precise balance of intrinsic genetic abnormality and extrinsic carcinogenic influence is extremely variable and thus perplexingly different in every patient.

Genetics is by strict definition the scientific study of heredity, so it is effectively the field of epigenetics that is of most interest to us in our studies of tumour biology and carcinogenesis. This is because it is particularly the latter which that aims to identify the detailed mechanisms by which individual genes bring about their recognisable or phenotypic effects and tries to determine how such pathways are distorted during cancer formation.

Modern concepts of carcinogenesis, of course, recognise the over-riding importance of molecular genetics. The mutations fundamental to cancer development are those that ultimately produce immortal cells that no longer respond to the normal intracellular and/or extracellular regulatory signals that control cell proliferation, differentiation and death.

Oral cancer and precancer

The annual estimated world incidence for combined intra-oral and oropharyngeal cancer is around 400 000 cases (making it the sixth most common cancer), with approximately 5000 new cases of oral cancer arising in the UK each year [1].

Over 95% of oral cancers are squamous cell carcinomas, originating from keratinocytes of the oral cavity's stratified squamous epithelial lining. They present most commonly as non-healing ulcerations due to tissue destruction, induration due to excessive keratin formation within tumour stroma, fixation to underlying tissues due to submucosal invasion and raised, everted tumour margins. Figure 3.2 shows the characteristic clinical appearance of a squamous carcinoma arising on the lateral tongue surface.

It is probably not surprising that oral epithelial cells are so vulnerable to cancer change, acting as they do as a defensive barrier against irradiation,

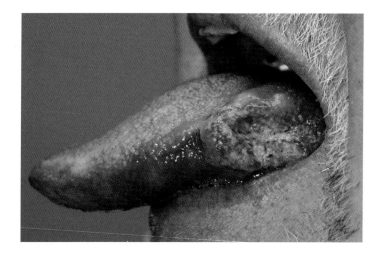

Figure 3.2 An exophytic squamous cell carcinoma arising from the lateral surface of the tongue showing classic raised, everted margins surrounding a central, cavitating ulceration.

pollutants in the air we breathe and carcinogens in the food and drink we consume. The fact that many carcinogens are ingested in large quantities, such as those in tobacco products and alcoholic beverages, only compounds the risk for the oral epithelium.

Essentially, a progressive stepwise mutation is believed to lead to a premalignant stage followed by malignant transformation, exhibited by increasing cellular dysregulation, growth abnormalities, cell immortality and ultimately invasive and metastatic malignant behaviour. The concept of an oral premalignant or pre-invasive state is based upon many longitudinal studies in which a number of identifiable oral precursor lesions have been seen to undergo malignant transformation, the observation that many premalignant lesions coexist with established carcinomas, and the fact that both premalignant and malignant disorders share common histopathological and/or biomolecular changes [2].

As we have previously discussed in Chapter 1, it is surprisingly difficult to determine accurate figures for either the overall incidence or prevalence of oral potentially malignant disorders, owing to considerable differences in the patient populations studied, variations in ethnicity and indigenous tobacco habits, and a lack of clarity for both clinical and histopathological definitions of lesions studied. Nonetheless, it is probably accepted that the estimated global prevalence runs somewhere between 2% and 3% [3].

Figure 3.3 summarises the various steps involved during oral carcinogenesis and the potential pathway that a keratinocyte may take through premalignancy to cancer. Cancer growth probably arises from clonal expansion and aberrant growth of a single stem cell or from a few tumour-initiating cells that acquire self-renewal capacity. Stem cells escape normal growth control, as a result of which they gain a significant growth advantage, allowing the development of an expanding clone which then displaces normal epithelial tissue. As the resulting lesion enlarges, additional genetic damage probably gives rise to numerous subclones. Subsequent clonal divergence and selection in such an inherently unstable field eventually gives rise to an invasive cancer [4].

As the tumour grows and develops, the genetic instability of the cancer may increase considerably, resulting in a heterogenous tumour cell phenotype, as discussed in the introduction above. Where there is a predominance of resistant, rapidly proliferating cells, this will clearly confer a significant advantage in terms of growth and survival.

Oral cancer cells will also be able to evade apoptosis by inactivation of apoptosis-inducing genes or by enhanced activity of anti-apoptosis genes

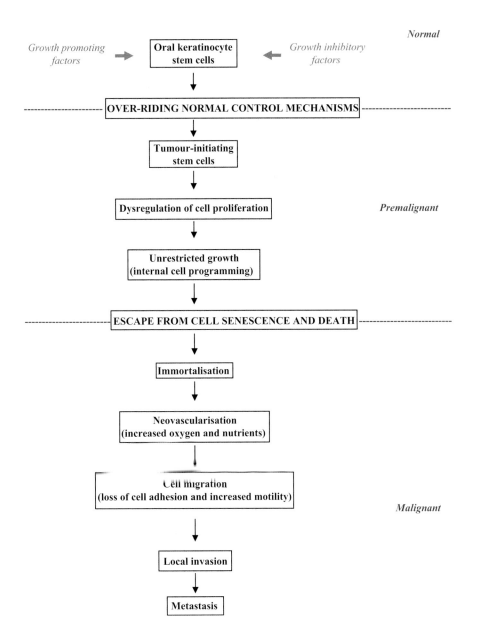

Normal

Premalignant

Malignant

Figure 3.3 Steps in oral carcinogenesis.

thereby allowing cell survival despite DNA damage, hypoxia and lack of nutrition. A variety of cell membrane factors, the anti-apoptotic action of BcL-2 proteins in mitochondria, and molecules within the cytosome – such as the inhibitor of apoptosis protein (IAP), survivin and ubiquitin – may all be involved in the evasion of apoptosis during carcinogenesis [5].

There also appears to be a significant increase in angiogenesis and overall vascularity in oral tissue during the transition from normal mucosa through increasingly dysplastic tissue to invasive carcinoma. Angiogenesis is known to be essential for tumour progression and metastasis and it is perhaps not surprising that increased angiogenesis accompanies both increased cell proliferation and decreased apoptosis as histological abnormalities increase in the mucosa [6,7].

What remains frustratingly difficult, however, is not only our inability to identify individual patients and oral lesions at risk of oral cancer change, but also our lack of any predictive ability to determine the nature and progression of this pathway to malignancy in the clinical situation.

The 'progression model' for oral cancer

Oral squamous cell carcinoma is thus regarded as a genetic disorder that develops from a series of stepwise mutations, sometimes spontaneously but more often than not due to some external carcinogenic influence. This leads to cellular changes that transform normal epithelium into invasive neoplasms. Fundamental to this process are alterations in the genes regulating cell division, cell cycle progression and DNA synthesis and repair. Promotion of oncogenes, inactivation of tumour suppressor genes and alteration of growth factor activity may all lead to abnormal regulation of cell proliferation, which as we have seen in Chapter 2, is recognised as a fundamental hallmark of carcinogenic change.

Oncogenes are derived from normal cellular gene products (proto-oncogenes) that have undergone mutation (point mutations, amplifications or rearrangement of DNA sequencing), conferring increased malignant potential. Tumour suppressor genes are believed to perform protective inhibitory roles at the cellular level, with mutation leading to loss of inhibitory control of cellular proliferation and loss of apoptosis (programmed cell death).

Box 3.2 summarises the many and varied proposed molecular mechanisms and resultant possible biomarkers involved in oral carcinogenesis. These involve multiple genetic and epigenetic events, including abnormalities in cell signalling, growth, survival, cell cycle control and angiogenesis, which together herald the progressive acquisition of a malignant phenotype [8,9]. It is important to emphasise that many of these processes overlap quite extensively and that they should not, therefore, be regarded as discrete mechanisms. The sequential order in which mutations arise is probably less important than their cumulative number and whilst the accumulation of such abnormalities may sometimes be due to random mischance, they are more commonly caused by environmental carcinogens, especially factors such as tobacco and alcohol.

Box 3.2 Mechanisms and markers of biomolecular disruption in oral carcinogenesis.

Oncogenes
- Signalling pathways:
    Epidermal growth factor
    Epidermal growth factor receptor
    Transforming growth factor alpha
- Transcription factors:
    Transcripting factor-activating protein
- Cyclins and cyclin-dependent kinases

Tumour suppressor genes
- p53
- Retinoblastoma protein

Genetic abnormalities
- DNA ploidy:
    Aneuploidy
    Allelic instability

- Chromosome abnormalities:
    Loss of heterozygosity
    3p 9p 13q 17p
- Mitochondrial mutation

Cell cycle disruption
- Cell proliferation:
    Labelling indices
- Cell differentiation:
    Cytokeratins
- Apoptosis:
    BcL-2
    Survivin

Loss of cell adhesion
- Annexins

- Syndecans

- Integrins

- Basement membrane components

Angiogenesis
- Vascular endothelial growth factor

- Nitric oxide synthase 2

Immortalisation
- Telomerase

- Retinoblastoma protein

- p16

Viruses
- Human papillomavirus 16

Prostaglandin synthesis
- COX-2 enzyme

Whilst molecular oncology has undoubtedly advanced our understanding of carcinogenesis, it is unfortunate that none of the biomarkers studied to date have been found to be of practical use in clinical practice. Laboratory studies of oral cancer and precancer tissue may analyse numerous molecular markers in an observational, cross-sectional way but do not, of course, facilitate clinical outcome data. They hence contribute little to improving our knowledge of the natural history of oral cancer disease.

Multistep progression from normal to dysplastic epithelium and eventual malignancy does, however, undoubtedly offer clinicians a therapeutic window of opportunity to intervene during carcinogenesis. The difficulty we have clinically is the ability to determine how far and how fast a precancerous lesion may be proceeding towards malignancy [10]. Later on during cancer progression multiple gene mutations are established, autonomous cell proliferation occurs, extracellular matrix is degraded, and invasion across epithelial basement membranes takes place leading to local tumour spread and eventual metastasis. By this stage, interventional treatment strategies can no longer control the disease process.

We now know that multiple gene pathways are involved in the progression from normal through dysplastic to cancer tissue, and that complex multiple gene analysis together with clinical outcome data will be necessary to produce any meaningful predictive analyses [11].

As none of these molecular markers are currently applicable in clinical practice, we still rely upon the recognition of phenotypic changes within the oral mucosa, seen histopathologically as epithelial dysplasia, the varying presence of cellular atypia and structural tissue dysmaturation that characterises potentially malignant disease. These important pathological features will be discussed in detail in Chapter 6.

Aetiology and risk factors

The aetiology of oral precancer and cancer is predictably multifactorial in nature (Box 3.3), although globally the most established risk factors are tobacco use (including smoking and chewing or snuff habits), excess consumption of alcohol and, particularly in South Asia, the use of the betel quid. Worldwide, 25% of oral cancers are attributed to tobacco use, 7–19% to alcohol abuse, 10–15% to nutritional deficiencies and 50% to betel chewing [12].

Box 3.3 Aetiology of oral cancer and precancer.

Inherent susceptibility
- Genetic predisposition

- Age

- Ethnicity

- Socioeconomic status

Tobacco use
- Smoking:
    Cigarette, cigar, pipe, bidi
    Reverse smoking
- Smokeless:
    Snuff dipping
    Tobacco sachets
    Tobacco chewing

Betel quid (pan) use
- Betel nut, slaked lime, tobacco and spices wrapped in betel leaf

---

Alcohol use
- Wine, beer, spirits
- Synergism with tobacco use

Diet and nutrition
- Low intake of fresh fruit and vegetables
- Iron and vitamin deficiencies
- High intake of processed meat products

Poor oral health and dental hygiene
- Possibly a promoting or co-factor in patients with heavy tobacco and alcohol use

Infective agents
- Human papillomavirus 16
- Candida
- Syphilis

Immunodeficiency
- Congenital
- Immunosuppression:
    Post-organ transplant
    Treating immune-mediated disease
- HIV infection and AIDS

Ultraviolet irradiation
- May lead to lip cancer

Other possible factors
- Mate drinking
- Khat chewing

AIDS, acquired immune deficiency syndrome; HIV, human immunodeficiency virus.

Many of these high-risk factors act synergistically, particularly tobacco and alcohol, whereby heavy drinkers and smokers have been estimated to have a nearly 40 times greater risk of developing mouth cancer than abstainers [1].

Tobacco

Whilst tobacco is primarily smoked worldwide, there are a number of specific populations whose tobacco habits include the use of either snuff (finely ground or cut tobacco leaves) or chewing tobacco (which comprises loose leaf products). Estimates suggest that the risk of oral cancer is nearly 3.5 times higher in smokers compared with non-smokers, with bidi smoking in India (which uses flaked tobacco rolled in a temburni leaf) being a particularly dangerous habit [13,14].

Tobacco products contain more than 70 known carcinogens, most importantly nitrosamines and polycyclic hydrocarbons such as benzo(a)pyrene. Whilst the latter are the most important carcinogenic agents in cigarette smoke, it is the nitrosamines that appear to cause most damage in unburnt tobacco [14]. A failure to metabolise and detoxify these carcinogens has been shown to lead to the adduction of active carcinogens to oral keratinocyte DNA [13].

Boyle et al. have recently reported on a number of changes observed in the buccal mucosa of smokers, including the overexpression of multiple genes involved in carcinogen metabolism, increased prostaglandin levels and a rise in Langerhans cells. Whilst such detailed genetic analyses become increasingly complex, the recognition of increased defensive action against carcinogens and a possible smoking-related change in mucosal immune function clearly highlight the increased risk of carcinogenesis in the oral mucosa of smokers [15].

Both oral cancer and precancer risk is related to both the intensity and duration of tobacco use, with patients who started to smoke before the age of 16 years appearing to be at a particularly enhanced risk [13]. Thus, the association between cigarette smoking and oral cancer is dose dependent with greater than 20 years smoking and more than 20 smoked cigarettes per day associated with a high risk of malignancy [12].

Importantly, however, the risk for patients who stop smoking is less than that of current smokers and there is a trend for decreasing risk with increasing number of years since quitting. Indeed, stopping smoking can effectively reduce the lifetime risk for patients of developing all upper aerodigestive tract cancers, although it may take up to 10 years for patients to reach the low-risk state of never smokers [13]. Similar observations have also seen established oral leukoplakic lesions regress and the incidence of new leukoplakias fall upon long-term tobacco cessation [13]. These are all very important epidemiological observations and should inform and motivate health care professionals to encourage quit attempts in their smoking patients.

Long-term tobacco smokers may show a number of clinically observable changes in the oral mucosal lining that can precede or accompany premalignant change and which effectively demonstrate underlying mucosal damage. It is very common, for example, to see a generalised erythema of the oral mucosa in smokers, especially within the floor of the mouth, and this is often accompanied by patches of hypermelanosis probably resulting from thermal and chemical irritation. These clinical features are illustrated in Figure 3.4.

Other commonly seen changes include stomatitis nicotina arising on the palatal mucosa and comprising irregular, thickened, white patches and scattered red spots due to swollen and inflamed minor salivary duct orifices (Figure 3.5). White patches, demonstrating hyperkeratosis histopathologically, may also be seen on the labial mucosa due to thermal damage from habitual cigarette holding habits. The classic clinical appearance of this is demonstrated in Figure 3.6.

Interestingly, whilst none of the above smoking-induced mucosal changes are regarded as potentially malignant in themselves, identification of such lesions on clinical examination should be regarded as clinical evidence that potential carcinogens are active within the mouth and are causing damage to the epithelial lining.

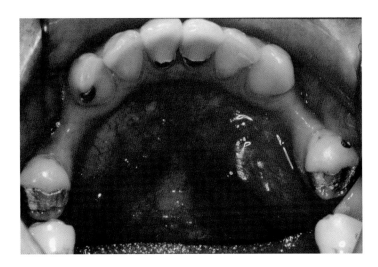

Figure 3.4 Erythematous floor of mouth tissue in a smoker, also showing patches of hypermelanosis due to tobacco-induced irritation.

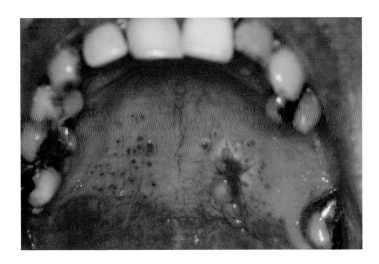

Figure 3.5 Stomatitis nicotina (smoker's keratosis) of the palatal mucosa, showing swollen, red minor salivary gland duct openings amongst a thick, white hyperkeratotic background. Note the healing incisional biopsy site laterally.

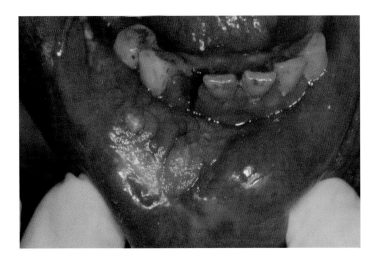

Figure 3.6 White patch arising on the labial mucosa due to thermal irritation from the habitual holding of a cigarette at this point. Histopathological examination showed hyperkeratosis only, but dysplasia may be seen in longstanding lesions.

Alcohol

Alcoholic beverages form a very heterogeneous group and contain variable percentages of ethanol (produced by carbohydrate fermentation) together with numerous other components including the potential carcinogens nitrosamine, acrylamide and polyphenols [12]. Ethanol is not in itself carcinogenic, but is metabolised to acetaldehyde which exerts multiple mutagenic effects on DNA. Alcohol also increases oral mucosa permeability, facilitating the passage of carcinogens through epithelial tissue more easily, and has a number of other systemic effects including hepatocellular damage, impaired detoxification, nutritional deficiencies and immunosuppression [16].

Whilst regular alcohol consumption is associated with increased oral cancer risk in a dose-dependent manner, the true aetiology is often obscured by simultaneous use of tobacco. People who consume alcohol but have never smoked may not have a significantly increased risk for oral carcinogenesis, although there may well be a trend for increasing oral alcohol intake to be associated with the observed increase in oral cancer in younger patients [12].

There is no clear evidence that any one particular type of alcohol, whether it be wine, beer or spirits, is more dangerous than another in terms of oral carcinogenesis. It is almost certainly the overall quantity of alcohol consumed that is the most important aetiological factor. In relation to oral precancer, Goodson et al. [16] observed that an alcohol intake of more than 28 units per week in smokers presenting with new oral dysplastic lesions in northern England, was associated with both a significantly increased severity of dysplasia at presentation and an increased risk of further dysplastic lesion development following treatment. This interesting observation not only supports the heightened risk associated with increased quantity of alcohol intake, but also emphasises the potentially damaging effect alcohol may have on pre-existing vulnerable and/or damaged oral mucosa.

Concerns have been raised intermittently through the years relating to alcohol-containing mouthwashes and oral cancer, but there are no reliable data to suggest this is a significant independent risk factor. Indeed, it is probably more likely that mouthwash users who develop oral cancer are actually heavy tobacco and alcohol consumers who use mouthwashes to disguise oral malodour.

Diet and nutrition

The consumption of fresh fruit and vegetables is associated with a reduced risk of oral cancer and appears similarly protective in precancer patients. Whilst this may reflect a generally better overall dietary and nutritional state, there may also be local effects modifying the oxidative state of transforming epithelial cells [17]. Thus, diets deficient in antioxidants (usually with a high fat and sugar content) may predispose to oral carcinogenesis. It must be remembered, however, that such epidemiological observations may be confounded by the fact that patients with poor diet often have heavy tobacco and alcohol consumption.

It has been estimated that nearly 90% of oropharyngeal cancers can be prevented by not smoking, decreasing alcohol intake and increasing consumption of fruit and vegetables [18]. This is a very powerful message indeed and certainly supports recent calls for multiple and repeated 'brief interventions' by health care professionals to encourage healthy living in at-risk patient groups.

There is no doubt that poor oral hygiene, tooth loss and periodontal disease are seen in many oral cancer patients, but whether this is a causal relationship or mere association remains unknown. It is certainly possible that chronic irritation from dental factors may act as promoters or co-factor in patients exposed to tobacco and alcohol. Thus there may be a polymicrobial mutagenic interaction within saliva, in which increased ethanol metabolism in chronic alcohol users increases the concentration of carcinogens such as acetaldehyde in the oral environment.

It is also known that oral cancer is much commoner in lower socioeconomic groups and in populations with high deprivation indices, who often have poor access to dental care, poorer diets and less healthy lifestyles [19].

The precise role of infective agents in the aetiology of oral cancer remains obscure, although certainly candidal infections and chronic conditions such as syphilis have been implicated in the past. Viruses have also been implicated in carcinogenesis and, with a possible sexually transmitted route involved, there is certainly some evidence that human papillomavirus infection (HPV16 in particular) may have a role in tonsillar and oropharyngeal tumours in younger patients [20].

A compromised immune system, whether due to a congential immunodeficiency or an acquired immunosuppression, may also predispose to oral carcinogenesis [21]. Acquired immunosuppression is most commonly due to drug therapy following organ transplant or to modulate an immune-mediated systemic disorder, or due to infections such as human immunodeficiency virus (HIV) and its resultant clinical presentation as acquired immuno deficiency syndrome (AIDS).

Of interest to note because of its misnomer, is a lesion termed 'hairy leukoplakia' which presents as irregular, raised, vertical white folds on the lateral borders of the tongue in HIV-infected patients. It is caused by an Epstein–Barr virus (EBV) infection and has no premalignant potential.

Genetic predisposition is also an important factor in oral carcinogenesis, as it is recognised that some patients (often those under the age of 45 years) who neither drink nor smoke develop precancer mucosal changes, presumably by accruing or inheriting DNA mutations by chance. Studies have shown that a family history of head and neck cancer increases the risk of developing disease, and gene polymorphism in genes encoding enzymes involved in the metabolism of tobacco and alcohol have also been seen.

Other patients with rare inherited cancer syndromes such as Fanconi's anaemia or xeroderma pigmentosum are also at higher risk of developing oral cancer [22].

There is no doubt that increasing age is an identifiable and probably somewhat independent risk factor for oral carcinogenesis. A not uncommon clinical presentation, for example, is that of an elderly female patient with no identifiable tobacco or alcohol risk factor behaviours who develops multiple precancer lesions on the oral mucosa (Figure 3.7). Lesions such as these often rapidly progress to invasive carcinomas with resultant poor clinical prognosis. Presumably, such potentially malignant disorders arise in inherently unstable oral mucosa with perhaps an age-related reduction in natural immune surveillance.

Interestingly, reviewing a number of studies on leukoplakia has shown no known identifiable cause for potentially malignant lesion development in

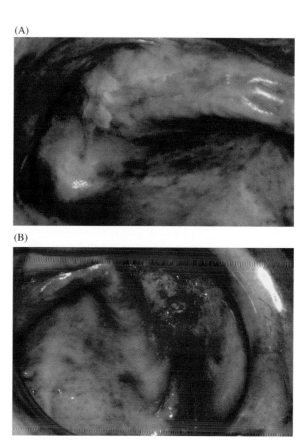

(A)

(B)

Figure 3.7 Multifocal presentation of potentially malignant lesions in an elderly, edentulous female patient.

4–27% of presenting patients, depending upon the precise population examined [3].

It is likely, therefore, that the path to invasive carcinoma development is a highly variable one, even within communities exposed to similar aetiological agents so that clinical outcomes for individual patients remain unpredictable. Whilst, as we have seen above, there is no doubt that overall the incidence of oral cancer and precancer increases with age, some patients in contrast display more rapid carcinogenesis and often at a much younger age than expected.

There also remains a fundamental uncertainty regarding exactly how many cancers are definitely preceded by clinically recognisable precancerous lesions and how many arise from apparently normal oral mucosa. This issue is somewhat clouded, of course, by the recognition that many oral cancers are diagnosed late in people who are irregular dental patients and who thus rarely attend for oral examination prior to their malignancy diagnosis.

Patient and risk factor profiling

The identification and stratification of individual patient risk factors in clinical practice thus remains elusive, but is a potentially vital component of comprehensive patient management. Indeed, the ability to characterise a risk profile package for each patient and their individual disease presentation would represent a 'gold standard' in clinical care.

Whilst the principal risk factors for precancer development and subsequent progression to cancer remain, of course, the use of tobacco and

Box 3.4   Risk factor profiling and oral precancer.

High risk
- Tobacco use
- Excess alcohol consumption
- Use of betel quid
- Predisposing genetic factors and inherent susceptibility
- Immunodeficiency
- Diet low in fresh fruit and vegetables
- Old age
- Marijuana use

Low risk
- Low socioeconomic status
- Poor oral health
- Use of shammah/toombak
- Human papillomavirus infection
- Candida albicans infection
- Diabetes mellitus

alcohol, Diajil et al. [23] reviewed 226 papers on oral cancer risk factors (published between 1982 and 2009). They stratified 14 different items according to possible risk severity, carcinogenicity and clinicopathological relevance. Box 3.4 summarises the resulting eight high-risk factors, which include tobacco and alcohol use, genetic predisposition and immunodeficiency, together with six lower risk factors such as socioeconomic status, oral health and infection.

It remains to be seen whether such individual patient risk profiling will ultimately prove useful in clinical practice, but it is highly likely that in the future all patient interventions will be tailored and targeted much more specifically than at present. Clinical outcome and disease progression following oral carcinogenesis cannot be predicted, which poses continuing management dilemmas for patient care. This, however, will be discussed in more detail in Chapter 8.

Summary

The pathway to invasive cancer development is a complex, multistep and multifactorial process. It is not always inexorable and indeed may well be reversible if early intervention in the process can occur to prevent further genetic mutation and disease progression. Whether this has a significant clinical implication for individual patients, allowing clinicians to intervene to stop the development of cancer, will be influenced by the efficacy of oral diagnosis and the recognition of potentially malignant conditions at the earliest possible stage.

The ability to identify which patients and which specific oral premalignant lesions are at greatest risk of cancer development is, of course, the ultimate goal of precancer management. These issues will be covered in detail in the next chapters of this book.

References

1. Warnakulasuriya S. Global epidemiology of oral and oropharyngeal cancer. *Oral Oncol* 2009; 45: 309–316.
2. Warnakulasuriya S, Johnson NW, van der Waal I. Nomenclature and classification of potentially malignant disorders of the oral mucosa. *J Oral Pathol Med* 2007; 36: 575–580.
3. Napier SS, Speight PM. Natural history of potentially malignant oral lesions and conditions: an overview of the literature. *J Oral Pathol Med* 2008; 37: 1–10.
4. Braakhuis BJM, Tabor MP, Kummer A, Leemans CR, Brakenhoff RH. A genetic explanation of Slaughter's concept of field cancerization: evidence and clinical implications. *Cancer Res* 2003; 63: 1727–1730.
5. Loro LL, Vintermyr OK, Johannessen AC. Cell death regulation in oral squamous cell carcinoma: methodological considerations and clinical significance. *J Oral Pathol Med* 2003; 32: 125–138.
6. Macluskey M, Chandrachud LM, Pazouki S. et al. Apoptosis, proliferation and angiogenesis in oral tissues. Possible relevance to tumour progression. *J Pathol* 2000; 191: 368–375.
7. Johnstone S, Logan RM. The role of vascular endothelial growth factor (VEGF) in oral dysplasia and oral squamous cell carcinoma. *Oral Oncol* 2006; 42: 337–342.
8. Molinolo A, Amornphimoltham P, Squarize C, Castilho RM, Patel V, Gutkind S. Dysregulated molecular networks in head and neck carcinogenesis. *Oral Oncol* 2009; 45: 324–334.
9. Smith J, Rattay T, McConkey C, Helliwell T, Mehanna H. Biomarkers in dysplasia of the oral cavity: a systematic review. *Oral Oncol* 2009; 45: 647–653.
10. Bosatra A, Bussani R, Silvestri F. From epithelial dysplasia to squamous carcinoma in the head and neck region: an epidemiological assessment. *Acta Otolaryngol (Stockh)* 1997; Suppl 527: 47–48.
11. Pitiyage G, Tilakaratne WM, Tavassoli M, Warnakulasuriya S. Molecular markers in oral epithelial dysplasia: a review. *J Oral Pathol Med* 2009; 38: 737–752.
12. Petti S. Lifestyle risk factors for oral cancer. *Oral Oncol* 2009; 45: 340–350.
13. Warnakulasuriya S, Dietrich T, Bornstein MM et al. Oral health risks of tobacco use and effects of cessation. *Int Dent J* 2010; 60: 7–30.
14. Warnakulasuriya KAAS, Ralhan R. Clinical, pathological, cellular and molecular lesions caused by oral smokeless tobacco – a review. *J Oral Pathol Med* 2007; 36: 63–77.
15. Boyle JO, Gumus ZH, Kacker A. et al. Effects of cigarette smoke on the human oral mucosal transcriptome. *Cancer Prev Res* 2010; 3: 266–278.
16. Goodson ML, Hamadah O, Thomson PJ. The role of alcohol in oral precancer: observations from a north-east population. *Br J Oral Maxillofac Surg* 2010; 48: 507–510.
17. Sandoval M, Font R, Manos M, Dicenta M, Quintana MJ, Bosch FX, Castellsague X. The role of vegetable and fruit consumption and other habits on survival following the diagnosis of oral cancer: a prospective study in Spain. *Int J Oral Maxillofac Surg* 2009; 38: 31–39.

18. Rugg-Gunn AJ. Nutrition, diet and oral health. *J R Coll Surg Edinb* 2001; 46: 320–328.

19. Greenwood M, Thomson PJ, Lowry RJ, Steen IN. Oral cancer: material deprivation, unemployment and risk factor behaviour – an initial study. *Int J Oral Maxillofac Surg* 2002; 32: 74–77.

20. Shillitoe EJ. The role of viruses in squamous cell carcinoma of the oropharyngeal mucosa. *Oral Oncol* 2009; 45: 351–355.

21. Scully C, Bagan J. Oral squamous cell carcinoma overview. *Oral Oncol* 2009; 45: 301–308.

22. Van der Waal I. Potentially malignant disorders of the oral and oropharyngeal mucosa; terminology, classification and present concepts of management. *Oral Oncol* 2009; 45: 317–323.

23. Diajil A, Goodson ML, Thomson PJ. Risk factors and oral precancer: developing a high/low risk profiling system. *Arch Otorhinolaryngol* 2010; 267 (Suppl 1): S39.

Clinical Presentation of Oral Precancer

Peter Thomson and Michaela L. Goodson

Oral Precancer: Diagnosis and Management of Potentially Malignant Disorders, First Edition. Edited by Peter Thomson.
© 2012 John Wiley & Sons, Ltd. Published 2012 by John Wiley & Sons, Ltd.

Introduction

Despite the tremendous advances seen in both molecular biology and also within the related sciences of genetics and epigenetics, the ability of individual clinicians to recognise and identify oral potentially malignant disorders, with their myriad of clinical presentations and subtle changes in mucosal appearance, remains absolutely fundamental to their accurate clinical diagnosis and subsequent management.

The term *oral precancer* was originally defined to include both discrete oral lesions and more widespread conditions, affecting not only the oral mucosa but also the patient in general, both of which demonstrate a variable and unpredictable potential to transform into invasive squamous cell carcinoma.

The new, preferred definition of *oral potentially malignant disorders* is probably a more encompassing term as it really implies a spectrum of morphological changes in oral mucosal tissue, many (but not all) observable clinically, which may show not only an increased potential for site-specific malignant transformation but also a risk of cancer development at other apparently clinically normal-looking oral sites.

This chapter is concerned with the clinical appearance of such potentially malignant changes in the mouth and the manner in which individual patients and disorders may present to clinicians. It is important to appreciate that, unfortunately, the vast majority of these conditions are symptomless and usually go unnoticed by patients until they have become quite extensive in size, have developed mucosal thickening or have become irritated in some way.

For practical purposes, then, this really means that most potentially malignant disorders will be found initially by dental practitioners during routine oral examinations, dental inspections or via oral health screening. Some patients, however, on eventually noticing symptoms may consult their general medical practitioner for advice regarding oral mucosal lesions. This is less common and can sometimes lead to delays in patient referral due to a lack of medical practitioners' experience in oral diagnosis.

Similarly problematic are the difficulties in identifying high-risk patients, the limitations of general population screening tests for oral cancer and the problems consequent upon the unpredictable and inconsistent natural history of oral precancer, all of which conspire to confound the diagnostic process. These issues will be explored in some detail in both this chapter and succeeding chapters of this book.

There remains little doubt, however, that a careful and methodical clinical examination by an experienced and alert clinician in an appropriate setting and with good lighting is the most reliable means of identifying oral lesions with the propensity for malignant transformation.

Clinical terminology

In Chapter 1 we listed a number of definitions relevant to the study of oral precancer. It is useful to review here and expand on some of these definitions, both those that have been used in the past but also and perhaps most importantly those currently favoured in the scientific literature to describe the varied clinical spectrum of oral precancer disease presentation. The wide range

Box 4.1 Clinical presentation of oral precancer disease.

Oral precancerous lesions
- Leukoplakia

- Erythroplakia

- Erythroleukoplakia

Oral precancerous conditions
- Immunosuppression

- Oral submucous fibrosis

- Lichen planus and lichenoid lesions

- Sideropenic dysphagia

- Discoid lupus erythematosus

- Actinic cheilitis

- Chronic hyperplastic candidosis (candidal leukoplakia)

- Syphilis

- Dyskeratosis congenita

of both lesions and conditions that comprise oral potentially malignant disorders are summarised in Box 4.1.

The term *oral precancerous (or premalignant) lesion* remains an extremely useful definition and was originally described by the World Health Organisation (WHO) in 1978 and referred to 'morphologically altered tissue in which cancer is more likely to occur than in its apparently normal counterpart'. This is very pertinent, as it highlights the significance of the epithelial tissue disorganisation and dysmaturation (encompassed by the histopathological term dysplasia) that is such an integral structural antecedent of neoplastic transformation.

Oral precancerous (or premalignant) conditions, in contrast to their discrete mucosal counterparts, however, are more generalized states associated with a significantly increased risk of cancer and include a range of systemic disorders in which oral manifestations are but one of many important disturbances.

A variety of other terms can be found in different publications through the years, all of which have been used to describe oral precancers, including: oral epithelial dysplastic lesions, epithelial precancer lesions, intraepithelial neoplastic lesions and oral or epithelial precursor lesions. This can lead to confusion for readers, especially when attempting to compare and contrast various clinical observations and analyses in published articles.

Thus, in 2007, a comprehensive review of both nomenclature and classification was undertaken following a workshop of the WHO Collaborating Centre for Oral Cancer and Precancer in the UK, and the new encompassing term, *potentially malignant disorders*, was proposed [1]. This term was felt to be particularly appropriate not only because not all precursor lesions inevitably transform into malignancy, but perhaps more significantly because of the recognition of field change carcinogenesis. Rather than discrete lesions and widespread conditions existing as separate entities there is a clear spectrum of potentially malignant disease, rendering the whole of the upper aerodigestive tract in such patients susceptible to malignant change.

We must therefore recognise that there exists within potentially malignant disorders a continuum of clinical presentations from discrete mucosal lesions through to more generalised or widespread precancerous conditions. Nonetheless, it remains helpful for the purposes of our description and analysis in this chapter to distinguish these various disorders in terms of lesions and conditions.

Precancerous (premalignant) lesions

Leukoplakia

Leukoplakia is by far the most common clinical presentation of oral precancer, accounting for 60–70% of all potentially malignant lesions [2,3]. The abnormal and/or increased keratin production characteristic of leukoplakia enhances tissue hydration by saliva resulting in the white appearance seen clinically in affected mucosa.

The classic definition of leukoplakia is thus of a 'white patch on the mucosa, which cannot be wiped off and which cannot be ascribed clinically or histologically into any other definable category'. Others have added that the white patch should not be associated with the use of any physical or chemical causation agent except tobacco, helping to emphasise the significance of tobacco in the aetiology of precancer disease [1].

Such an unqualified 'diagnosis by exclusion' is somewhat unsatisfactory, however, as it fails to emphasise the significant risk of dysplastic change and its consequent malignant potential within such lesions. The principal distinguishing feature of leukoplakia from other oral keratoses (white patches with thickened keratin layers) is indeed the histopathological recognition of epithelial dysplasia, and these important pathological features of leukoplakia will be discussed in more detail in Chapter 6.

Numerous attempts to refine the diagnosis of leukoplakia have therefore taken place, including the 2005 amended WHO clinical definition of 'white plaques of questionable risk, having excluded (other) known diseases or disorders that carry no increased risk for cancer'. This is useful as it emphasises the risk of carcinoma development, which is of course the principal concern in diagnosing and managing such lesions.

There are, however, no clear histological requirements for a white mucosal lesion to fulfil this definition and leukoplakia remains, as it always has been, very much a clinical descriptive term.

Oral leukoplakia has a reported prevalence of 2–3% worldwide and is significantly more common in males although, as we have seen, females are also affected [4]. In the developed nations, leukoplakias are usually seen in middle-aged or elderly patients especially between the fifth and seventh decades. However, there is no doubt that in the European setting we have experienced a demonstrable and significant increase in the number of younger patients presenting with leukoplakic lesions.

Leukoplakia is six times more common amongst smokers than non-smokers and can affect any part of the oral cavity and oropharynx. However, the buccal mucosa worldwide and the floor of the mouth and ventrolateral tongue in Western populations are probably the commonest anatomical sites affected [2,3]. The precise site of leukoplakia development in a population is probably influenced to a large extent by the preferred local tobacco habit. Tobacco smoking is thus associated particularly with leukoplakia on the buccal mucosa, ventral tongue surfaces and the floor of the mouth, whilst buccal lesions alone are commonly seen where tobacco chewing habits predominate, with palatal lesions seen uniquely in reverse smokers. The latter is a particular habit in which the lighted end of a coarse cheroot (or chutta) is held inside the mouth, particularly seen in females from a number of Indian coastal districts.

Schepman et al. (2001) reviewed 166 oral leukoplakia patients in a Netherlands population and noted that whilst the floor of the mouth was the commonest overall site of origin for leukoplakia in smoking patients, male smokers also showed a propensity for lesions to appear at the labial commissure and buccal mucosal regions. In contrast, leukoplakias arising on the lateral borders of the tongue were most commonly seen in non-smoking females. Interestingly, there appeared to be no clear explanations why such specific gender differences should exist [5].

There are a number of factors, however, that are readily defined and identifiable in patients and which may contribute to determining the site of origin of individual leukoplakia lesions. These are summarised in Box 4.2. In addition, Table 4.1 lists the varying clinical appearance and presentation of a number of different leukoplakic lesions that may arise in response to a range of smokeless tobacco habits carried out worldwide. These were discussed in Chapter 3 and include different forms of oral snuff, various tobacco chewing habits and the use of tobacco products mixed with areca nut or lime and applied to the oral mucosa.

Box 4.2 Factors influencing the site of oral leukoplakia presentation.

Oral mucosa
- Type and extent of mucosal keratinsation
- Mucosal permeability
- Epithelial cell proliferative activity

Oral environment
- Salivary pooling
- Mucosal irritation
- Oral hygiene

Tobacco habit
- Tobacco smoking
- Cigarette placement/habitual cigarette holding
- Reverse smoking habits
- Smokeless tobacco use

Smokeless tobacco habit	Geographical location	Oral sites affected	Clinical appearance
Snuff	Sweden, USA	Anterior maxillary Labial sulcus	Diffuse, wrinkled, grey/white leukoplakia
Chewing tobacco	USA	Anterior mandibular Buccal/labial sulcus Alveolus	Corrugated, raised leukoplakia
Betel quid	South Asia	Posterior mandibular Buccal sulcus	Fissured leukoplakia Erythroleukoplakia Multiple lesions Oral submucous fibrosis
Toombak	Sudan	Buccal/labial mucosa Floor of mouth	Verrucous leukoplakia
Shamma	Yemen	Gingiva	Verrucous leukoplakia
Khaini	Nepal	Anterior mandibular Buccal/labial sulcus	Fissured erythroleukoplakia
Nass	Central Asia, Pakistan	Mandibular Buccal/labial sulcus	Wrinkled leukoplakia

Table 4.1 Aetiology and clinical presentation of oral smokeless tobacco lesions.

It is clear that site-specific lesion presentation is directly linked to the type of smokeless tobacco used and the preference to habitually place the product at a particular intra-oral location. Lesions tend to evolve with prolonged use of the tobacco product, varying from an initial superficial wrinkling of the mucosa through white/grey discolouration to thickened, white, deeply furrowed or verrucous lesions. Whilst some authors have sought to distinguish smokeless tobacco lesions from their smoking-related leukoplakic counterparts, they are probably all best regarded as part of the overall spectrum of oral potentially malignant disorders [6].

It is also important to appreciate that the many differences seen in quoted figures for overall leukoplakia incidence and prevalence undoubtedly exist not only because of variations in geographic location but also because of differences between types of patients studied. This is especially so for the distinction between general community-based population studies compared with specialist hospital clinic studies. The pattern and presentation of precancer disease in the latter will be highly and selectively influenced by both patient referral patterns and clinician interest and awareness.

Once fully established as a mucosal lesion, leukoplakia may appear clinically in a variety of different forms and it is important that clinicians are aware of these many and often subtle variations (Box 4.3). What remains unclear, however, is how long it takes individual leukoplakic lesions to become clinically apparent, nor is it certain how many lesions may actually change or alter their appearance with time.

Nonetheless, a number of general observations can be made. Homogeneous leukoplakias are defined as flat and uniformly white throughout the entire lesion, appearing as either feint patches (Figure 4.1) or as much thicker lesions, sometimes resembling a coating of paint (Figure 4.2). On other occasions, whilst remaining uniform, the leukoplakia may exhibit a ribbed or rippled appearance, sometimes compared to the appearance of the ebbing tide at the sea shore. This is shown presenting on the posterior buccal mucosa in Figure 4.3.

Box 4.3 Clinical appearance of leukoplakia.

Homogeneous
- Feint
- Thick
- Ribbed/rippled (ebbing tide)

Non-homogenous
- Warty/thickened
- Nodular

Mixed homogenous/non-homogenous
Verruciform
- Simple verrucous
- Proliferative verrucous leukoplakia

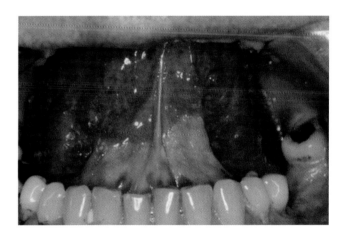

Figure 4.1 Feint, homogeneous leukoplakia arising in the anterior floor of the mouth.

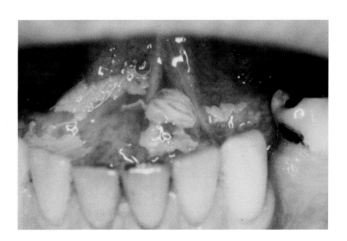

Figure 4.2 Thick, paint-like leukoplakia irregularly distributed on the floor of the mouth.

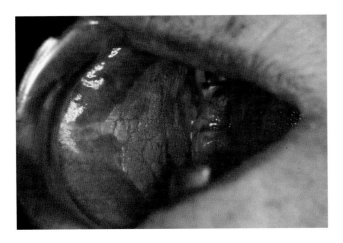

Figure 4.3 Wrinkled or 'ebbing tide' leukoplakia arising on the posterior buccal mucosa.

Non-homogeneous leukoplakia can appear as irregular, widespread, thickened areas as seen arising in the floor of the mouth and ventral tongue in Figure 4.4 or as more localised nodular lesions as illustrated on lateral tongue mucosa in Figure 4.5. Mixed patches of homogenous and non-homogenous lesions are also observed, usually when widespread areas of mucosa are affected such as in the buccal mucosa of Figure 4.6.

Whilst some leukoplakias present as small, distinct lesions, other patients may exhibit extensive and widespread mucosal disease. These range from large, feint, diffuse leukoplakias to multiple lesions presenting at distinct oral sites

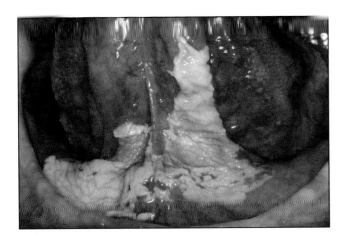

Figure 4.4 Irregular, widespread and thickened leukoplakia arising in the ventral tongue and spreading onto the floor of the mouth.

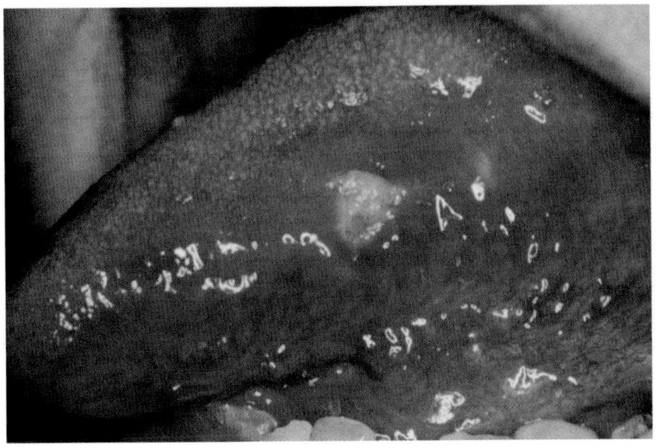

Figure 4.5 Localised, nodular leukoplakia on the lateral border of the tongue.

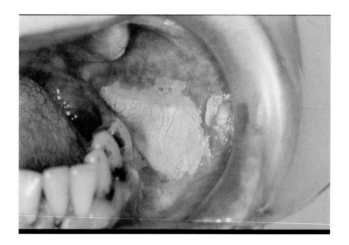

Figure 4.6 Mixed, non-homogeneous leukoplakia arising on the buccal mucosa and comprising feint, wrinkled ('ebbing tide') and nodular components.

separated by normal-looking mucosa. The patient who presents with multiple, synchronous, leukoplakic lesions is probably representative of a specific and distinct precancer disease entity and a detailed description of this will be presented later in this chapter.

The term *verrucous leukoplakia* has often been applied to a particular clinical presentation of a non-homogeneous lesion that differs from flat homogeneous leukoplakia by its extremely wrinkled, corrugated and warty texture. It may be clinically indistinguishable from verrucous carcinoma, which is a rare, primarily locally invasive variant of oral squamous cell carcinoma [7] Figure 4.7 demonstrates a particularly florid example of a verrucous leukoplakia extending from the mandibular alveolus into the floor of the mouth in an elderly edentulous patient.

Proliferative verrucous leukoplakia (PVL) is a rare but more recently recognised and important subgroup of leukoplakic lesions. These lesions are slow growing and progressive and appear as expanding, fissured, exophytic and warty-looking white patches, characterised by multifocal presentation, resistance to treatment and a high rate of malignant transformation, often in the absence of identifiable dysplastic features on previous biopsy. Whilst PVL lesions usually present initially as slowly expanding solitary, asymptomatic, white lesions these inevitably progress over time as multiple similar lesions occur, ultimately progressing into large, warty masses. Although lesions may be removed surgically, there is a high rate of both recurrence and new lesion development [8].

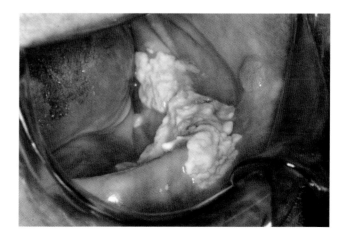

Figure 4.7 Extensive verrucous leukoplakia arising on the mandibular alveolus and extending into the floor of the mouth and buccal sulcus. Note the papillomatous buccal lesion nearby.

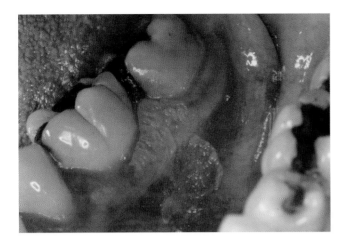

Figure 4.8 Relatively localised, proliferative verrucous leukoplakia involving the mandibular buccal gingiva and alveolar mucosa and extending into the buccal sulcus.

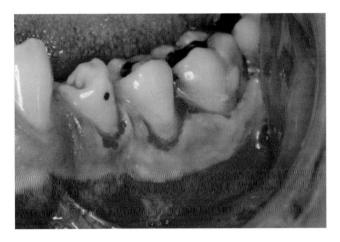

Figure 4.9 A more widespread proliferative verrucous leukoplakia extending along the attached buccal gingiva of the posterior mandibular teeth.

PVL lesions most frequently present on the gingiva, and the alveolar and buccal mucosae, typically arising in patients in their sixth or seventh decades and more commonly in women than men. The precise aetiology of PVL is obscure and, unlike others forms of oral leukoplakia, there appears to be no strong association with the use of tobacco and alcohol. Figure 4.8 shows a relatively localised PVL lesion arising on the mandibular buccal gingiva, whilst Figure 4.9 illustrates a much more widespread presentation involving most of the attached gingiva. The lesions shown in Figure 4.10, however, are more

(A)

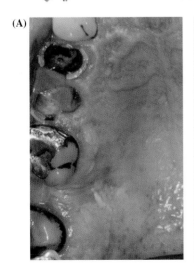

(B)

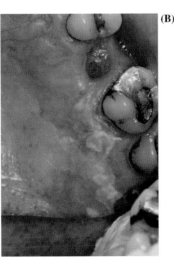

Figure 4.10 (A, B) Extensive proliferative verrucous leukoplakia involving the palatal gingiva bilaterally and extending diffusely over the palatal mucosa.

Box 4.4 Characteristic clinicopathological features of proliferative verrucous leukoplakia.

- Slow growing, progressive, multifocal leukoplakia

- Mainly affects female patients >60 years old

- Primarily arises on gingiva, buccal and alveolar mucosae

- No strong association with tobacco or alcohol use

- Hyperkeratosis, verrucous hyperplasia and a lymphocytic 'lichenoid' infiltrate may be seen histopathologically

- Resistant to all treatment, with recurrence common following surgical excision

- Malignant transformation occurs in 70–100% of cases

characteristic of the typical multifocal appearance of proliferative verrucous leukoplakia involving both the gingiva and palatal mucosa.

The diagnosis of PVL is based upon the clinical appearance of lesions together with a number of tissue architectural disturbances seen histopathologically. The latter features vary depending upon the stage of the disease, so that initial hyperkeratosis (usually without the presence of epithelial dysplasia) is followed by verrucous hyperplastic change leading on to verrucous carcinoma and then the development of invasive squamous cell carcinoma. An intense lymphocytic infiltrate may also be observed in PVL lesions obscuring the basement membrane and epithelial–connective tissue interface and possibly leading to confusion with lichen planus and lichenoid lesions, which are conditions described later in this chapter [8]. Malignant transformation rates for PVL varying from 70% to 100% have been quoted in recent papers, which clearly emphasizes the high clinical risk associated with these lesions. Signs suggesting transformation to malignancy include rapid growth of the verrucous patch, the appearance of red or erosive areas and induration [9].

Box 4.4 summarises a number of important clinicopathological characteristics of PVL, some of which may help to distinguish this condition from conventional tobacco-associated oral leukoplakia.

For all oral leukoplakic lesions it is advisable in the clinical situation to record not only the specific appearance of individual leukoplakias, but also to document their precise anatomical location, whether the lesions are single or part of a multiple lesion presentation, and to measure both the size of the lesion and the overall extent of involved oral mucosa. Additional information to document carefully in each affected patient includes suspected aetiological agents, such as tobacco smoking, abuse of alcohol and the use of smokeless tobacco products and betel or areca nut use.

Differential diagnosis It is relatively straightforward to distinguish leukoplakia from transient white patches that are easily wiped off the oral mucosal surface and arise from the accumulation of epithelial debris or inflammatory exudates, such as those seen in acute pseudomembranous candidosis (Figure 4.11). However, there are a number of persistent non-dysplastic white lesions that may be mistaken for potentially malignant lesions. Table 4.2 lists these white patches and highlights features that may help to distinguish them from leukoplakia.

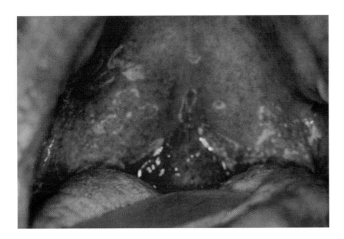

Figure 4.11 Soft, white, removable exudate signifying an acute pseudomembranous candidosis, here arising on the soft palate following steroid inhaler use.

Condition	Clinical features
Hereditary (genodermatoses)	
Oral epithelial (white sponge) naevus	Shaggy, folded and ill-defined soft, white lesions appearing in childhood or adolescence (autosomal dominant inheritance)
Leukoedema	Translucent, milky white buccal mucosa (normal variant)
Pachyonychia congenita	White, opaque thickening of buccal, lingual and labial mucosae
Tylosis	White plaques on buccal mucosa
Follicular keratosis	Rough, whitish papules or plaques on gingiva, tongue and palate
Hereditary benign intraepithelial dyskaryosis	White, spongy, macerated buccal lesions
Chronic trauma	
Frictional keratosis	Dense, white, roughened plaques adjacent to a source of chronic irritation
Chemical trauma	Thickened, white patches with oedema, necrosis and sloughing
Thermal trauma	White plaques on buccal mucosa, tongue, palate and lips

Table 4.2 Differential diagnosis of leukoplakia

Erythroplakia

Erythroplakia appears less commonly in the oral cavity than leukoplakia and may be seen as a bright or fiery red, velvety patch, with either a smooth, depressed or granular surface, which is usually well defined from surrounding normal-looking mucosa. (The older term 'erythroplasia', originally coined by Queyrat and applied to a similar lesion on the glans penis, is infrequently used nowadays.) In contrast to leukoplakia, oral erythroplakic lesions are often symptomatic, so that patients themselves may become aware of their presence and often complain of areas of mucosal sensitivity or soreness.

Prevalence figures for erythroplakia vary between 0.02% and 0.83%, mainly presenting in middle-aged and elderly patients with no specific gender preference [7]. Alcohol, smoking and candidal infection are regarded as important aetiological factors. Lesions are usually solitary and, although any site in the oral cavity may be affected, the floor of the mouth is a particularly common site (Figure 4.12).

Erythroplakia has long been considered to have the greatest potential for malignant transformation. Histopathologically, lesions show atrophic epithelium, hence the red colouration visible clinically, and often exhibit severe dysplasia or carcinoma in situ. In some cases, microinvasive or early invasive

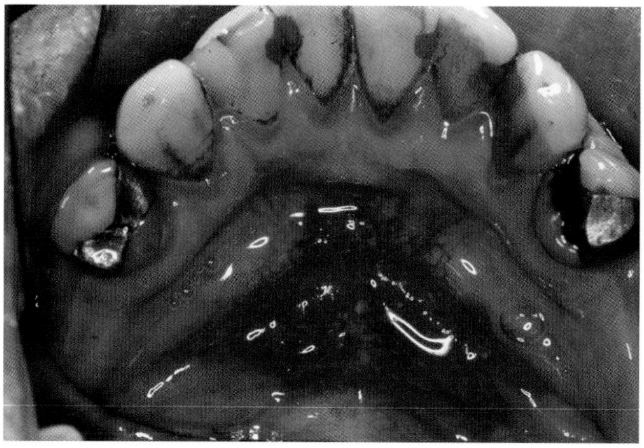

Figure 4.12 Erythroplakia presenting in the midline of the anterior floor of the mouth.

Box 4.5 Differential diagnosis of erythroplakia.

Inflammatory/immune mediated
- Desquamative gingivitis
- Erosive lichenoid lesions
- Pemphigoid
- Reiter's disease
- Hypersensitivity reaction

Infection
- Erythematous (atrophic) candidosis

Trauma
- Purpura

Tumours
- Haemangioma
- Kaposi's sarcoma

squamous cell carcinoma may already be present. As a result, most erythroplakias will ultimately undergo malignant transformation and they are thus regarded as very high-risk lesions.

Differential diagnosis Box 4.5 lists a number of other mucosal conditions that may give rise to red oral mucosal patches and which should be distinguished from true erythroplakia.

Erythroleukoplakia

This lesion, which is a combination often of nodular leukoplakic patches on a background of eryrthroplakic change (sometimes referred to as 'speckled

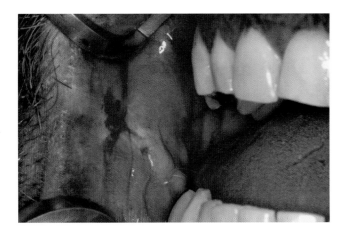

Figure 4.13   An erythroleukoplakic lesion arising in the labial commissure region and extending inwards towards the buccal mucosa. Biopsy confirmed the diagnosis of chronic hyperplastic candidosis, associated with the presence of severe epithelial dysplasia.

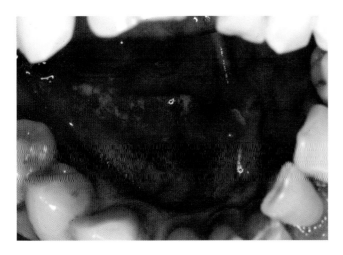

Figure 4.14   Erythroleukoplakia ('speckled leukoplakia') arising in the floor of the mouth.

leukoplakia') is also much less common than leukoplakia. It may arise at any site in the oral cavity but is particularly common at the labial commissures, where it may be associated with a chronic candidal infection (Figure 4.13), or on the floor of the mouth (Figure 4.14). Erythroleukoplakias also tend to be high-risk lesions and have a much greater tendency to develop malignancy than homogeneous leukoplakias.

High-risk clinical appearance

From the point of view of clinical presentation, a number of features have come to be recognised as important in raising concern of an increased risk of malignant transformation within an oral precancer lesion. These features are summarised in Box 4.6.

Potentially malignant disorders arising in the floor of the mouth, ventrolateral tongue and the retromolar and faucial regions thus appear to be most at risk, whilst it is recognised that erythroplakias and erythroleukoplakias carry a higher risk than leukoplakias. Non-homogeneous or nodular leukoplakic lesions may also be at greater risk of developing malignancy than their homogeneous counterparts.

Box 4.6 Clinical features associated with a high risk of malignant transformation.

Lesion site
- Floor of mouth
- Ventrolateral tongue
- Retromolar trigone
- Pillars of fauces

Clinical appearance
- Erythroplakia
- Erythroleukoplakia
- Proliferative verrucous leukoplakia
- Non-homogeneous leukoplakias
- Multiple lesion disease

Lesion behaviour
- Rapid increase in size
- Appearance of red areas or erosions
- Pain, bleeding, ulceration
- Development of induration or fixation

A rapid increase in lesion size, the appearance of reddened areas, erosions or ulcerations, and the onset of induration and fixation are all highly suspicious signs of squamous cell carcinoma arising in oral precursor lesions and the presence of any of these should raise concern. Figure 4.15 illustrates localised ulceration, induration and fixation arising within leukoplakia on the ventrolateral border of the tongue and, in this case, signifying the development of an invasive carcinoma.

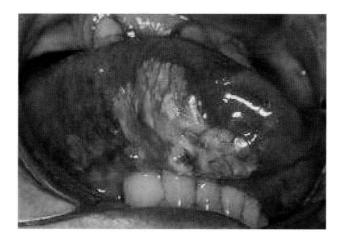

Figure 4.15 Localised ulceration, induration and fixation arising within leukoplakia on the ventrolateral tongue. This is the beginning of an invasive squamous cell carcinoma.

It is important, however, to stress than there are no definitive or consistently reliable clinical predictors of malignancy and that the above descriptors are part of a continuum of clinical appearances that often merge together. The malignant transformation of precursor lesions will be discussed in more detail in Chapter 8.

Precancerous (premalignant) conditions

There is little doubt that between them leukoplakia, erythroplakia and erythroleukoplakia account for, by far, the most commonly occurring oral potentially malignant disorders worldwide. Nonetheless, there are a number of more generalised conditions in which cancers may arise within the oral cavity and oropharynx and it is important to recognise that they may also have a significant role as potentially malignant disorders.

Immunosuppression

Probably the commonest precancerous conditions seen in UK and European populations are those in which patients suffer from immunodeficiency or immune suppression. This may arise in congenital immunodeficiency cases but is seen most commonly in modern clinical practice in patients on prolonged use of immunosuppressive drugs following organ transplant. Acquired immune deficiency syndromes in human immunodeficiency virus (HIV) infected patients may also predispose to oral dysplastic lesions. More rarely, oral dysplasia with a high risk of malignancy may be seen in patients suffering from or with a history of graft versus host disease following bone marrow transplantation.

Lesions in immunocompromised patients appear predominantly as leukoplakias in the clinical situation and can arise at any intra-oral site, although the lips and labial commissures are most commonly affected. Such lesions may rapidly progress to squamous carcinomas, as illustrated in the labial mucosa of Figure 4.16. It is important to recognise that multiple lesions are extremely common in immunocompromised patients and they may arise both synchronously and metachronously.

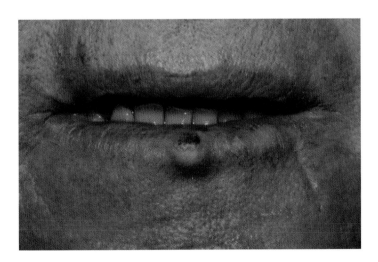

Figure 4.16 Squamous cell carcinoma arising on the labial mucosa of an immunocompromised (post-transplant) patient. Note the scar laterally following a wedge excision of a previous carcinoma at this site.

Lichen planus and lichenoid lesions

This is a particularly interesting and quite common condition and controversy has existed for many years in the literature about whether oral lichen planus should be considered a potentially malignant disorder or not.

Classic lichen planus is a chronic, inflammatory, mucocutaneous disorder, almost certainly of multifactorial origin – including genetic, psychological, infectious and autoimmune aetiologies – in which T lymphocytes accumulate immediately subjacent to altered, keratinised, acanthotic or atrophic oral epithelium. Hyperkeratosis gives rise to white striae, plaques or nodules on the mucosa, whilst severe epithelial atrophy or liquefactive basal cell degeneration produces diffuse red lesions, erosions or bullae on affected mucosae.

The buccal mucosa is most often involved with lichenoid lesions, which appear both symmetrically and bilaterally (Figure 4.17). Whilst a white, lace-like pattern is the commonest presentation on the buccal mucosa, erosive lesions are sometimes predominant and may give rise to large areas of denuded epithelium (Figure 4.18).

The tongue, gingiva, palate and lips are also frequently affected by lichen planus. Unlike other forms of leukoplakia, which are rare on the tongue dorsum, lichenoid lesions often appear in a widespread manner as illustrated in Figures 4.19 and 4.20.

Overall, most authors accept that there may be a small risk of malignant transformation in lichen planus, although this is probably less than 1 %. Whilst atrophic and erosive forms have traditionally been felt to be at higher risk, owing to the decreased barrier presented to potential carcinogens, it seems that clinical appearance alone is an unreliable predictor of cancer development, with malignancy also observed to arise from plaque-type lesions. The area of mucosa

(A)

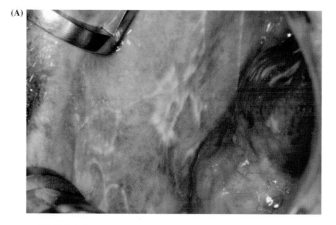

(B)

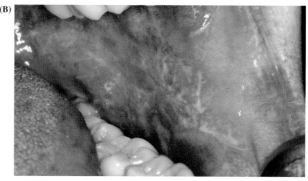

Figure 4.17 Lichen planus, classically presenting as reticular white patches bilaterally on the buccal mucosa (A). (B) A localised erosion in the mucosa inferiorly near the occlusal plane.

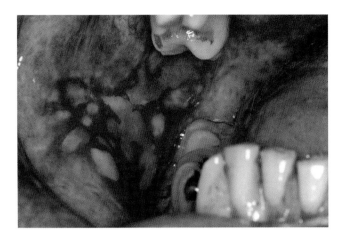

Figure 4.18 An extensive, erosive lichenoid lesion affecting the buccal mucosa.

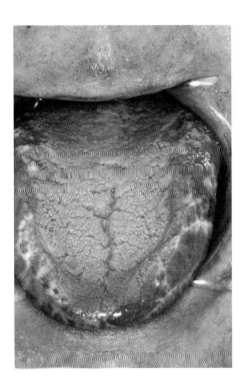

Figure 4.19 Widespread lichen planus affecting the dorsum and bilateral mucosal surfaces of the tongue.

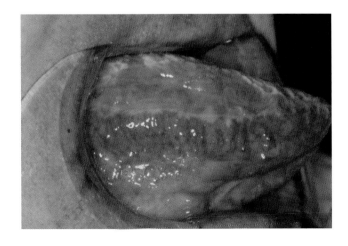

Figure 4.20 Although an unusual site for oral leukoplakia, lichenoid lesions may often appear in a widespread distribution on the dorsum of the tongue. This view demonstrates a clear delineation from the normal-looking lateral and ventral tongue mucosa.

affected by lichenoid change may also be relevant, with extensive mucosal disease affected by 'field cancerisation' effects. Another complicating factor in categorising the risk of malignant transformation in lichen planus is the recognition of a separate category of oral lichenoid lesions or reactions that are clinically indistinguishable from idiopathic lichen planus. Aetiologically, they may be triggered by hypersensitivity reactions to drug therapy, topographically to old amalgam restorations, in chronic graft versus host disease or as unclassified lichenoid lesions lacking one or more characteristic features of lichen planus, such as bilateral presentation [10].

The absence of strict diagnostic criteria to differentiate between lichen planus and lichenoid lesions confounds the diagnostic process, placing great emphasis on the judgement and experience of individual clinicians. Incisional biopsy of lichenoid lesions for histopathological assessment and to exclude the presence of epithelial dysplasia or invasive carcinoma is thus recommended for all cases. Where widespread lichenoid lesions affect multiple oral sites, it is advisable to carry out 'field mapping' biopsies to characterise as accurately as possible the disease distribution and to determine the precise location of any dysplastic element.

It is difficult to comment precisely on the malignant potential of individual lichenoid lesions, but it is probably best to consider them all as potentially malignant. Where possible, patient management should include the recognition and elimination of any aetiological factors.

Some authors have advocated the use of the histopathological term lichenoid dysplasia to describe the presence of a band-like lymphocytic infiltrate beneath the dysplastic epithelium [11]. Anecdotal clinical reports have suggested that these lesions, which clinically may appear indistinguishable from other lichenoid eruptions, have a particularly high risk of malignant transformation, although no consistent results exist in the literature to confirm this. Whilst some researchers have suggested that it is lichenoid dysplasia and not lichen planus that should be categorised as potentially malignant, others have emphasised that these conditions are unlikely to be distinct entities but rather to form part of a continuum of alterations in epithelial cell growth, differentiation and proliferation that ultimately may predispose to malignant transformation.

Regardless of clinical appearance, it is likely to be the histological appearance of dysplasia within lichenoid lesions that is the most important diagnostic factor and such lesions should thus be regarded as primarily dysplastic, high-risk potentially malignant disorders. It may be that the intense inflammatory cell infiltrate in the immediate subepithelial tissue demonstrates an enhanced immune response to antigenically altered dysplastic epithelial tissue.

Oral submucous fibrosis

This is an unusual chronic, insidious disorder in which fibrosis of the mucosa of the oral cavity, oropharynx and upper third of the oesophagus may occur. It can present with a burning sensation exacerbated by spicy food, progressing to mucosal vesiculation and blanching. Thereafter the mucosa becomes leathery in texture and vertical fibrous bands appear in the cheeks and faucial pillars and often extending to encircle the lips. Late changes can include distortion of the uvula and further woody changes to the buccal mucosa and tongue. Figure 4.21

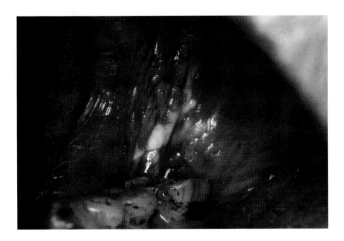

Figure 4.21 Oral submucous fibrosis affecting the buccal mucosa. Note the presence of mucosal atrophy and erosion, diffuse leukoplakia and mucosal ridging due to thickening of collagen fibres in the submucosa.

demonstrates the classic clinical appearance of affected buccal tissues with leukoplakic patches, mucosal erosions and ridging due to thickened collagen fibres in the submucosa.

Oral submucous fibrosis is predominantly found in Southeast Asia and is well recognised as a potentially malignant disorder. The main cause is thought to be the use of betel quid, an areca nut mixture with slaked lime wrapped in a betel vine leaf, which is held in the mouth. Heavy consumers of betel may consume 20–30 quids daily and the habit of betel quid chewing is often acquired in childhood. Clinically, the teeth are stained dark red or brown by a dye extracted from the nut by the lime (Figure 4.22) and at the site of quid placement there is often mucosal erythema and sometimes erythroplakia or leukoplakia (Figure 4.21). Fibrosis and hyalinisation occurs in the lamina propria, resulting in a loss of vascularity, mucosal pallor and subsequent atrophy of the overlying epithelium.

The atrophic epithelium is thought to predispose to the development of squamous cell carcinoma in the presence of carcinogens, with an annual malignant transformation rate of approximately 0.5%. Unfortunately, there are no established markers to identify which individuals may be predisposed to the disorder, we cannot reliably establish the risk of malignancy in affected patients, and there are no clearly effective treatment strategies [7,12].

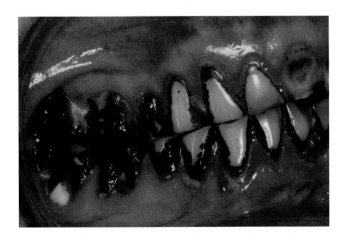

Figure 4.22 Extensive red-brown staining of the dentition and marked attrition as a result of betel chewing in an oral submucous fibrosis patient.

Sideropenic dysphagia

Sideropenic dysphagia (Plummer–Vinson or Patterson–Kelly–Brown syndrome) is actually quite a rare condition that usually presents in middle-aged females and comprises glossitis, dysphagia (due to proximal oesophageal web formation) and iron deficiency anaemia. Although primarily associated with the development of postcricoid carcinoma, this disorder can also give rise to dysplastic lesions in atrophic oral mucosa.

Discoid lupus erythematosus

This is a chronic, autoimmune condition that affects females more commonly than males and presents with scaly red patches on the facial skin, often symmetrically across the nose and cheeks in a butterfly pattern (Figure 4.23). Intra-oral lesions occur most commonly on the buccal mucosa and usually appear as discoid areas of erythema or ulceration surrounded by white keratotic borders and clinically may resemble lichen planus or erythroplakia. A classic stellate-shaped buccal mucosal lesion is shown in Figure 4.24. Malignant transformation is known to occur and often affects lesions presenting on the labial and buccal mucosa.

Actinic cheilitis

This is a clinically descriptive term for ulcerative and sometimes crusted lesions found partly or fully covering the vermilion border of the lower lip. Often seen in elderly men and usually due to prolonged or excessive exposure to ultraviolet light, the histopathological spectrum varies from hyperkeratosis with or without epithelial dysplasia through to early squamous cell carcinoma. Precise rates of malignant tranformation are unknown due to a lack of studies with cohorts of untreated patients [8].

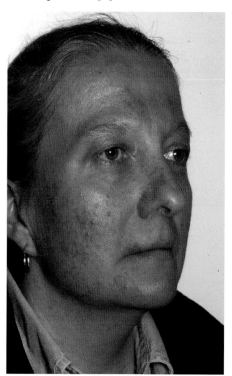

Figure 4.23 A female patient with discoid lupus erythematosus, demonstrating an erythematous, scaly rash over the cheeks and nose. Often this has the classic 'butterfly' appearance involving both cheeks and the bridge of the nose.

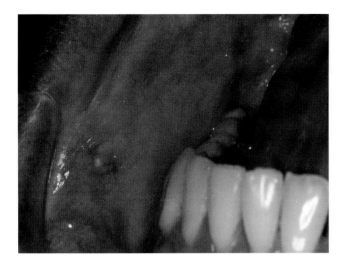

Figure 4.24 An oral mucosal lesion in discoid lupus erythematosus, illustrating a characteristic star-shaped erythematous patch on the buccal mucosa, with peripheral radiating white striae.

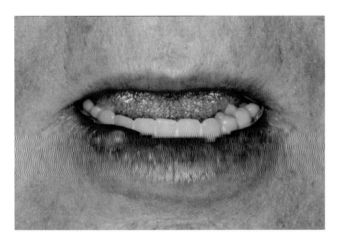

Figure 4.25 Early changes associated with actinic cheilitis affecting the lower labial mucosa. There is oedema of the lip together with feint, white mucosal changes reminiscent of a lichenoid appearance. Thickening and erosion are seen towards the right side of the lip.

Similar lesions may be seen on the lips in immunocompromised patients and the differential diagnosis for actinic cheilitis should also include lichen planus, which can arise on the labial mucosa and may resemble the early stages of ultraviolet damage clinically. Figure 4.25 demonstrates some of the early mucosal changes seen in actinic cheilitis

Chronic hyperplastic candidosis (candidal leukoplakia)

These lesions present as dense, opaque and nodular leukoplakias, often triangular in shape and commonly seen symmetrically positioned bilaterally at the labial commissures (Figure 4.26). These lesions are particularly common in heavy smokers and tobacco may well be the principal aetiological agent. Sometimes the presence of erythematous patches within the lesions produces a speckled appearance.

Histopathologically, areas of hyperkeratosis and acanthosis together with patches of atrophic epithelium account for the speckled leukoplakic appearance. Candidal hyphae invade the parakeratin at right angles reaching as far as the prickle cell layers. Reactive cellular atypia, possibly in response to carcinogens generated by *Candida* interacting with the effects of tobacco, may be reversible following antifungal therapy but in other cases may progress to definite epithelial dysplasia.

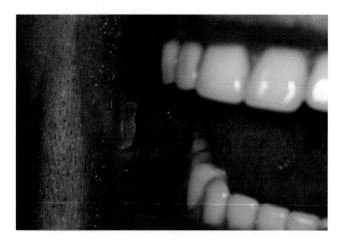

Figure 4.26 Chronic hyperplastic candidosis presenting as an irregular, non-homogeneous leukoplakic plaque at the labial commissure of an edentulous patient.

Whilst it remains unclear whether chronic hyperplastic candidosis is primarily a dysplastic leukoplakia secondarily infected by *Candida* or a primary candidal infection that leads to secondary dysplasia, there is no doubt that there is a significantly high risk of malignant change, especially in patients who continue to smoke.

Syphilis

Very rarely these days, inadequately treated patients with syphilis may present in the tertiary stages of their disease with oral leukoplakia particularly affecting the dorsum of the tongue. These widespread, feint, leukoplakic lesions exhibit an extremely high risk of malignant transformation. The precise aetiology of syphilitic leukoplakia remains unclear, but may be related to both epithelial atrophy and a chronically impaired immune surveillance system. Figure 4.27 shows the typical appearance of both mucosal atrophy and widespread leukoplakia seen in the lingual mucosa of a patient with tertiary syphilis.

Dyskeratosis congenita

Dyskeratosis congenita is a rare, probably recessively inherited, condition affecting males and manifesting with oral leukoplakia, dystrophy of the nails, greyish-brown skin pigmentation and haematological abnormalities including

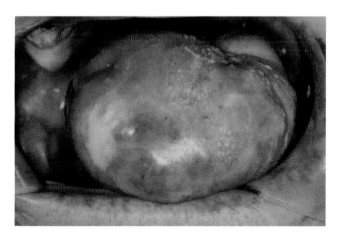

Figure 4.27 Mucosal atrophy, together with ill-defined, widespread feint leukoplakia, characteristic of the appearance of the lingual mucosa in tertiary syphilis.

immunodeficiency. Oral lesions initially appear as vesicles or ulcerations on the tongue and buccal mucosa in childhood, followed by the accumulation of white patches of necrotic epithelium, leading to reddening of the mucosa and finally by 20–30 years of age the establishment of erosive leukoplakia, which has a high malignant potential.

Multiple lesion disease

Whist the vast majority of patients with oral potentially malignant disorders exhibit single lesion disease, a very important subgroup of patients, reportedly affecting between 3% and 24% of oral precancer cases, actually present with multiple oral lesions. In these patients extensive areas of mucosa can exhibit dysplastic change. Figure 4.28 shows the widespread and variable appearance of multiple potentially malignant lesions affecting the floor of the mouth, mandibular alveolus and buccal mucosa in a longstanding smoker.

We have already seen that the modern concepts of carcinogenesis that evolved from the classic field cancerisation work of Slaughter emphasise the existence of molecularly altered preneoplastic fields from which multiple oral lesions, both synchronously and metachronously, can develop [13,14]. A number of possible explanations to explain multiple lesion disease presentation have been proposed through the years, and these are summarised in Box 4.7 [15].

Whether multiple lesion disease represents a distinct presentation in patients more susceptible to DNA damage and multiple genetic abnormalities due to enhanced tobacco and alcohol exposure, or is just an evolution of precancer

(A)

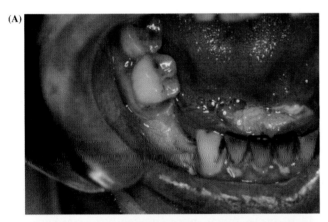

(B)

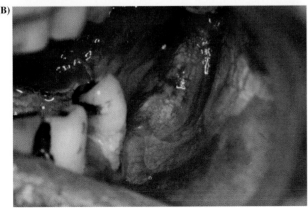

Figure 4.28 Multiple lesion disease showing mandibular alveolar and floor of mouth leukoplakia (A), together with erythroleukoplakia in the left mandibular alveolus and buccal leukoplakia (B).

Box 4.7 Possible origins of multiple lesion disease.

• *Preconditioning*:	Field change during organogenesis generates a large area of preconditioned 'unstable' epithelium
• *Early simultaneous mutations*:	An early genetic event occurring simultaneously in a group of epithelial cells, thus priming them for subsequent genetic mutation
• *Polyclonal origin*:	Multiple, distinct genetic alterations occurring in different clonally independent cells
• *Monoclonal expansion*:	Single genetic event leading to clonal expansion and lateral spread throughout the epithelium creating a large preneoplastic field

disease over time remains to be seen. However, a number of distinct clinico-pathological differences between single and multiple disease patients have been observed through the years.

Saito et al., for example, in 1999 reviewed the features of 99 localised and 12 widespread leukoplakias in a Japanese population presenting over a 20-year period [16]. They observed that whilst the gingiva and tongue were the commonest sites for localised lesions, widespread leukoplakias were most commonly seen to arise on the gingiva and buccal mucosa. Although no significant differences were found between the degrees of dysplasia seen in localised compared with widespread lesions, the rate of developing carcinoma was noted to be much higher in patients with widespread leukoplakia. Saito et al. thus postulated that different aetiological mechanisms may account for the two distinct types of presentation and suggested further studies would be beneficial.

Thomas et al. (2003) reviewed 115 Indian patients with multiple oral premalignant lesions and found that tobacco chewing habits in particular (although interestingly not tobacco smoking) and alcohol drinking were the strongest risk factors for multiple lesion development. A high vegetable intake in the diet was believed to have a protective effect against multiple lesion disease, although a similar effect for fruit intake was not seen [17].

More recently, we compared the clinicopathological features of 78 patients from northeast England presenting with single dysplastic oral lesions with 18 multiple lesion cases. Few significant differences were seen with respect to patient age, gender, smoking or alcohol status, but multiple lesions were observed to occur much more frequently in smokers who consumed little in the way of both fruit and vegetables [18]. Distinct differences were also seen in terms of clinical presentation. Whilst overall, most precancer lesions appeared clinically as homogeneous leukoplakias, erythroleukoplakia and ulcerated lesions were more likely to present as discrete, single lesions. Single lesions were also seen to occur more commonly on the floor of the mouth and ventrolateral tongue, whilst multiple lesions were more prevalent on the buccal mucosa. The soft palate, retromolar regions and tongue dorsum also exhibited a higher involvement in multiple lesion disease and at these sites lesions often exhibited a non-homogeneous or erythroplakic appearance [18].

Although both severe dysplasia and higher cell proliferative activity was seen in single lesions, with multiple lesions showing mainly mild dysplasia and lower proliferation, there was a tendency for more significant dysplasia to be found in all lesions arising in the soft palate and faucial regions.

There also appears to be a higher incidence of carcinoma development in multiple lesion patients, probably reflecting a more widespread mucosal instability. Indeed multifocal or widespread precancer should be regarded as a marker for increased cancer risk not just within the oral cavity but throughout the entire upper aerodigestive tract [16,18,19]. Malignant transformation and the development of invasive carcinoma will be discussed in more detail in Chapters 8 and 9.

Patients presenting with multiple lesions may thus represent a distinct clinical group at higher risk of persistent disease and malignant transformation. Strategies for managing multifocal disease are thus much more challenging than those required for single lesion disease and involve field mapping biopsies, regular and careful clinic review and targeted interventional laser surgery [20]. These important clinical management techniques will be discussed in more detail in Chapter 7.

Summary

Oral potentially malignant disorders may present clinically as localised mucosal lesions, or as part of a more widespread multifocal disorder. The classically described lesions and conditions probably form more of a continuum of precancer disease, which can affect the whole upper aerodigestive tract in susceptible patients. A persistent clinical management problem is the early identification of symptomless mucosal changes in an 'at-risk' population that rarely attends for regular oral and dental examination.

The ability to identify precancer change and facilitate early intervention to prevent oral carcinogenesis depends upon thorough and accurate oral examination by trained clinicians. Whether this can be supplemented by population screening, targeting of high-risk individuals and the use of advanced diagnostic techniques will be discussed in more detail in the next chapter.

References

1. Warnakulasuriya S, Johnson NW, van der Waal I. Nomenclature and classification of potentially malignant disorders of the oral mucosa. *J Oral Pathol Med* 2007; 36: 575–580.
2. Thomson PJ, Wylie J. Interventional laser surgery: an effective surgical and diagnostic tool in oral precancer management. *Int J Oral Maxillofac Surg* 2002; 31: 145–153.
3. Hamdah O, Thomson PJ. Factors affecting carbon dioxide laser treatment for oral precancer: a patient cohort study. *Lasers Surg Med* 2009; 41: 17–25.
4. Petti S. Pooled estimate of world leukoplakia prevalence: a systematic review. *Oral Oncol* 2003; 39: 770–780.
5. Schepman KP, Bezemer PD, van der Meij EH, Smeele LE, van der Waal I. Tobacco usage in relation to the anatomical site of oral leukoplakia. *Oral Dis* 2001; 7: 25–27.
6. Warnakulasuriya KAAS, Ralhan R. Clinical, pathological, cellular and molecular lesions caused by oral smokeless tobacco – a review. *J Oral Pathol Med* 2007; 36: 63–77.

7. van der Waal I. Potentially malignant disorders of the oral and oropharyngeal mucosa: terminology, classification and present concepts of management. *Oral Oncol* 2009; 45: 317–323.

8. Bagan J, Scully C, Jimenez Y, Martorell M. Proliferative verrucous leukoplakia: a concise update. *Oral Dis* 2010; 16: 328–332.

9. Gandolfo S, Castellani R, Pentenero M. Proliferative verrucous leukoplakia: a potentially malignant disorder involving periodontal sites. *J Periodontol* 2009; 80: 274–281.

10. van der Waal I. Oral lichen planus and oral lichenoid lesions; a critical appraisal with emphasis on the diagnostic aspects. *Med Oral Patol Cir Bucal* 2009; 14: E310–314.

11. Krutchkoff DJ, Eisenberg E. Lichenoid dysplasia: a distinct histopathologic entity. *Oral Surg Oral Med Oral Pathol* 1985; 60: 308–315.

12. Kerr AR, Warnakulasuriya S, Mighell A.J. et al. A systematic review of medical interventions for oral submucous fibrosis and future research opportunities. *Oral Dis* 2011; 17 (Suppl 1): 42–57.

13. Slaughter DP, Southwick HW, Smejkal W. Field cancerization in oral stratified squamous epithelium: clinical implications of multicentric origin. *Cancer* 1953; 6: 963–968.

14. Thomson PJ. Field change and oral cancer: new evidence for widespread carcinogenesis? *Int J Oral Maxillofac Surg* 2002; 31: 262–266.

15. Dakubo GD, Jakupciak JP, Birch-Machin MA, Parr RL. Clinical implications and utility of field cancerization. *Cancer Cell Int* 2007; 7: 2.

16. Saito T, Sugiura C, Hirai A. et al. High malignant transformation rate of widespread multiple oral leukoplakias. *Oral Dis* 1999; 5: 15–19.

17. Thomas G, Hashibe M, Jacob BJ, Ramadas K, Mathew B, Sankaranarayanan R, Zhang Z-F. Risk factors for multiple oral premalignant lesions. *Int J Cancer* 2003; 107: 285–291.

18. Hamadah O, Goodson ML, Thomson PJ. Clinicopathological behavior of multiple oral dysplastic lesions compared with that of single lesions. *Br J Oral Maxillofac Surg* 2010; 48: 503–506.

19. Lee JJ, Hong WK, Hittlelam W.N. et al. Predicting cancer development in oral leukoplakia: ten years of translational research. *Clin Cancer Res* 2000; 6: 1702–1710.

20. Thomson PJ, Hamadah O. Cancerisation within the oral cavity: the use of 'field mapping biopsies' in clinical management. *Oral Oncol* 2007; 43: 20–26.

5 Diagnostic Methods

Peter Thomson and Michaela L. Goodson

Oral Precancer: Diagnosis and Management of Potentially Malignant Disorders, First Edition. Edited by Peter Thomson.
© 2012 John Wiley & Sons, Ltd. Published 2012 by John Wiley & Sons, Ltd.

Introduction

Diagnosis refers to the act, or perhaps more appropriately, the art of identifying the precise nature and significance of a disease process presenting in a patient. This is clearly a highly unsatisfactory definition in terms of oral precancer, however, because most potentially malignant lesions are unfortunately asymptomatic for a long period during their evolution and exhibit inconsistent or unpredictable natural histories. Similarly, patients are often totally unaware of their condition and, due to the fact that many patients with risk factors do not attend regularly for dental or oral examination, abnormal mucosal appearance may remain undiscovered for many months or even years.

In most cases, the diagnosis of precancer is based upon the recognition of a suspicious-looking lesion by an experienced clinician during a routine oral examination and then ascribing an appropriate term to the lesion. This is then usually followed by an incisional biopsy of the lesion to facilitate histopathological assessment and thus confirmation of the clinical diagnosis.

Histopathological examination also allows assessesment of any significant tissue disorganisation and dysmaturation changes, which if present are categorised into varying degrees of epithelial dysplasia. We will examine the important and fundamental role of these pathological descriptors of oral precancer disease in some detail in the next chapter of this book.

Unfortunately, however, neither clinical appearance nor histopathological classification offers a reliable prognosis for individual patients or their lesions. Indeed, if clinical examination proves unsuccessful in discovering suspicious lesions, both potentially malignant states and frankly invasive tumours may all go unrecognised.

Oral examination remains the most commonly applied assessment, but there is no doubt that by itself it has limited value as a method for ensuring detection of all suspicious lesions. A number of diagnostic aids have thus been developed to try to improve detection. These include vital tissue-staining techniques, enhanced light-based detection and imaging systems and exfoliative cytology. Whilst still largely in the development phase, they all show potential as screening tools, but their application and accuracy of use requires further research in order that a precise role for each diagnostic test can be identified.

In this chapter we will review the role of population screening for oral precancer, outline the importance and efficacy of conventional visual examination of the oral mucosa, and discuss the potential use of diagnostic aids or adjuncts in precancer diagnosis and management.

Screening

Screening is defined as a structured health care intervention that is designed to detect disease at latent or asymptomatic stages, thereby interrupting disease progression or facilitating cure. On the face of it, this would seem highly appropriate for oral precancer but despite the apparent simplicity and appropriateness of a visual oral examination as a screening tool, there is actually little evidence to support oral cancer population screening [1]. This is due to:

- The difficulty in attracting high-risk patients to attend for screening.

- The presence of many benign mucosal abnormalities that confound the diagnostic process.

- The varied clinical appearance of potentially malignant precursor lesions.

- The recognition that many precancer lesions exist in clinically normal-looking mucosa.

It is also problematic that there is a lack of agreed treatment protocols for managing oral precancer lesions following their discovery and a lack of good evidence to show that subsequent preventive and therapeutic approaches markedly improve long-term patient outcomes.

Targeted screening of individuals deemed to be at high risk of carcinogenesis may offer opportunities for risk factor modification and prevention. However, case finding – which is the application of a diagnostic test to a patient who already presents with abnormal signs or symptoms in order to establish a diagnosis – and opportunistic testing of high-risk groups are probably of more greater value as tools in oral precancer diagnosis and in facilitating early interventional strategies [2].

It is well recognised that patients who smoke and drink excessively and who are thus most at risk of oral cancer are also likely to have poor diets, come from lower socioeconomic groups and are least likely to access medical services or to attend their dentist for regular oral examination. The problem therefore remains how to encourage such individuals to attend for clinical assessment. In addition there are real practical questions as to how, when and to whom they should present themselves for examination.

It would seem logical that the clinical responsibility for early identification of oral mucosal changes and the recognition of the potentially malignant nature of suspicious oral lesions should rest ultimately with dental practitioners. However, a recent study involving primary care practitioners in northern England raised concerns about the lack of a rigorous and systematic approach amongst many dentists towards not only the recognition of suspicious oral signs and symptoms, but also to the actual detection and management of established potentially malignant lesions [3]. A similar problem was also noted in relation to the difficulties facing general dental practitioners in identifying early cases of oral cancer and the perceived failure of the conventional axiom that recommends that dentists should screen all their patients for oral cancer at every routine check up [4].

The real dilemma is that public awareness of oral cancer and its associated risk factors remains generally low in most populations. It seems clear that improving public awareness of oral cancer and precancer and targeting education towards 'at-risk' individuals to alert them to potential signs and symptoms of early-stage disease together with a greater emphasis on prevention should now be the major priorities for future oral health care.

Clinical examination techniques

Careful and thorough mucosal examination by a trained clinician in a good light remains the standard method for identifying suspicious oral lesions. In view of the comments above, all clinicians should be encouraged to improve the quality of their routine oral mucosal examinations. It is also very important that the clinician adheres to a regular routine and is methodical in inspecting every region of the oral cavity to avoid missing abnormalities.

A useful method commences with examination of the anterior floor of the mouth and ventral tongue and then moves backwards bilaterally along the lateral tongue surfaces, inspecting both the lingual mucosa and then the

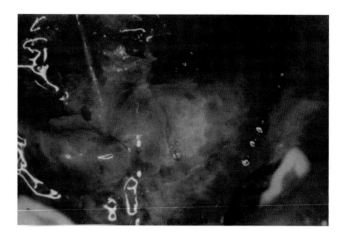

Figure 5.1 Leukoplakia of the floor of the mouth just extending onto the ventral tongue, as revealed during an anterior oral cavity examination.

posterior floor of the mouth. Figure 5.1 shows leukoplakia arising in the floor of mouth, whilst Figure 5.2 demonstrates probable frictional hyperkeratosis extending along lateral tongue surfaces and corresponding to the occlusal line of the teeth.

The patient is then asked to protrude the tongue forwards as far as they can and then to point their tongue tip first to the right and then to the left side to visualise the posterior tongue and tongue base (Figure 5.3). Whilst the tongue dorsum remains an unusual site for potentially malignant disease it is very important to obtain good visualisation of the posterolateral lingual mucosa, where precancer commonly presents. In an alternative technique, the clinician can gently manipulate and manoeuvre the tongue with a damp swab but this is uncomfortable and many patients are intolerant, which can lead ultimately to a poorer quality examination.

The lingual mandibular gingiva and retromolar areas are then examined, aided by the use of a dental mirror. This can be a difficult area to visualise but, as illustrated in Figure 5.4, many potentially malignant lesions arise at these sites and can remain hidden unless specifically looked for.

The patient is then asked to say 'Ah' which allows direct visualisation of the faucial pillars, tonsils and soft palate. In many cases tongue depression with a spatula or mirror may improve the view, but some patients are actually quite intolerant of this manoeuvre, resulting in a poorer examination. Figure 5.5 illustrates a diffuse leukoplakia covering most of the soft palate mucosa.

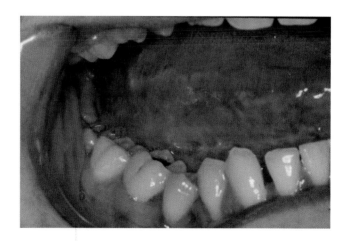

Figure 5.2 Inspection of the lateral tongue mucosa showing frictional hyperkeratosis along the occlusal line.

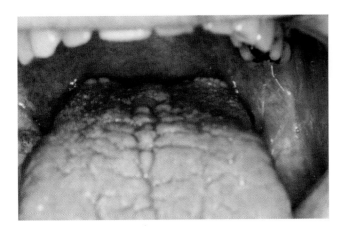

Figure 5.3 Direct visualisation of the posterior third of the tongue is best achieved by asking the patient to protrude their tongue as far forwards as possible.

The hard palate and palatal gingiva are best seen by direct visual inspection (Figure 5.6), as is the buccal mucosa. The latter should be examined bilaterally starting posteriorly at the pterygomandibular raphe and finishing anteriorly by careful inspection of both labial commissures and then the upper and lower lip mucosa and vermilion borders. Figure 5.7 demonstrates an extensive buccal mucosal lichenoid lesion and Figure 5.8 illustrates a feint leukoplakia arising at the labial commissure and extending backwards along the buccal mucosa.

Finally, the patient is asked to close the teeth together and all labial and buccal gingival surfaces are examined. It is surprisingly easy to miss subtle leukoplakic lesions on gingival surfaces, as shown in Figure 5.9, unless careful examination is performed.

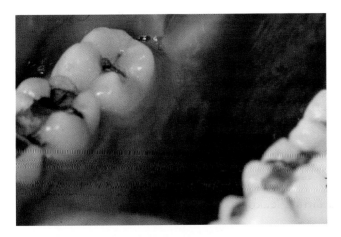

Figure 5.4 The lingual retromolar region, here showing a localised erythroleukoplakia, is best visualised by dental mirror examination.

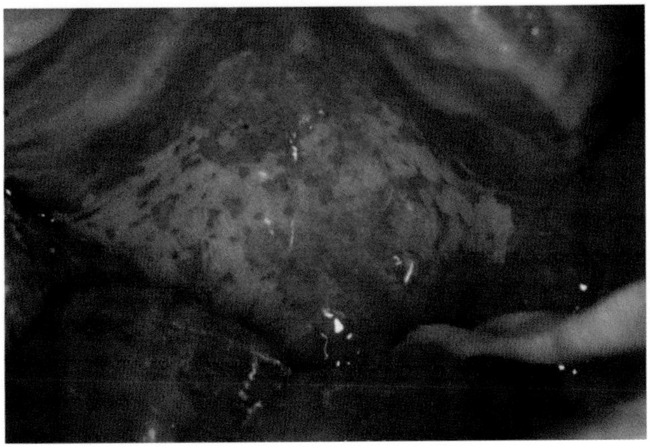

Figure 5.5 The soft palate is usually best visualised by both tongue depression and instructing the patient to say 'Ah', here illustrating a diffuse leukoplakia.

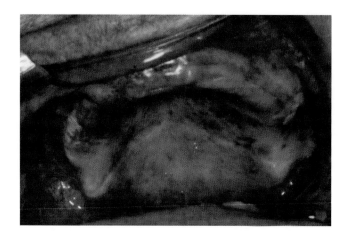

Figure 5.6 Direct visualisation of the edentulous maxillary alveolus and hard palate showing bilateral alveolar leukoplakic lesions.

If a suspicious mucosal lesion is found, its location, size, morphology and surface characteristics should be recorded. Lesions should then be gently palpated with gloved fingers, which helps determine whether they are soft and mobile or of more sinister nature – appearing firm, indurated, fixed to underlying structures and friable or haemorrhagic. Leukoplakic lesions should be further assessed to see if they can be wiped away by careful use of a damp swab, in which case the diagnosis may well be that of an acute pseudomembranous candidosis. Sometimes, feint or inconsistent lesions can be visualised better and finer details revealed by gentle application of a dry swab to remove overlying moisture on the mucosal surface.

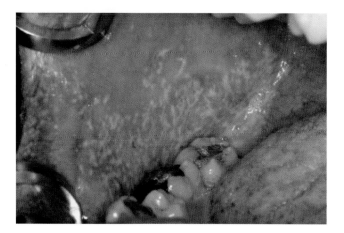

Figure 5.7 Buccal mucosa examination revealing an extensive lichenoid lesion.

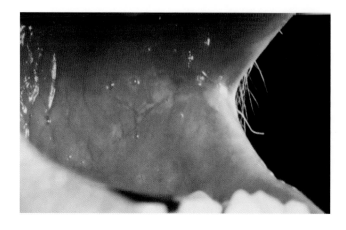

Figure 5.8 Feint leukoplakia arising in the labial commissure region and extending backwards along the buccal mucosa.

(A)

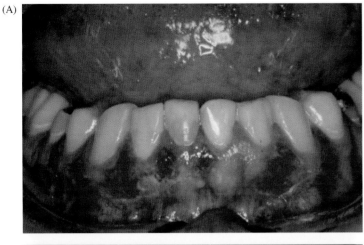

(B)

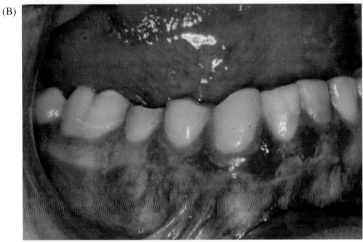

Figure 5.9 Mandibular gingiva demonstrating widespread feint leukoplakia at both labial (A) and buccal (B) sites.

It is important that the findings of clinical examination are recorded accurately and concisely. Some clinicians will record the lesion diagrammatically or enter it on a mouth map (Figure 5.10) to demonstrate both size and location. Others prefer to photograph lesions and include these records in patients' notes, which is particularly helpful in hospital practice where patients may not always be reviewed by the same clinician at each clinic visit.

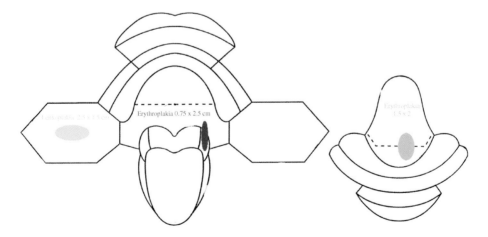

Figure 5.10 A mouth map used to record the site, shape, size and clinical description of potentially malignant lesions.

Box 5.1 Investigation of the oral precancer patient.

- Patient history:
    Identification of risk factors
    Recognition of medical conditions predisposing to precancer

- Clinical examination:
    Visual inspection of oral mucosa
    Palpation of oral lesions
    Wiping away pseudomembranous conditions

- Clinical investigations: oral swab for microbiological assessment

- Blood tests:
    Full blood count
    Ferritin, vitamin B_{12}, folate
    Urea and electrolytes
    Random blood glucose
    Liver function tests

- Clinical photography

- Incisional biopsy and histopathological assessment

Following thorough visual inspection, the clinician will then have to determine which further investigations are required. Box 5.1 summarises the investigations that may be required to establish a complete diagnosis for a newly presenting oral precancer patient.

All cases will certainly require an incisional biopsy for histopathological examination. It is important to select a specific site for biopsy that includes the most representative and/or clinically severe-looking region, together with the lesion margin and adjacent normal-looking tissue. Whilst incisional biopsies are vital diagnostic tests, they only provide a provisional result because they may not always be entirely representative of the nature of the whole lesion [5].

A specific diagnostic problem is posed by patients who present with multiple lesions or pan-oral disease. Such multifocal disease may affect up to 24% of patients with oral cancer and visualisation of the true extent of the disease, particularly where there is extensive involvement of the posterior oral cavity and pharynx, can be extremely difficult. In these cases, it is useful to consider a more detailed examination under anaesthesia to facilitate a comprehensive inspection. Multiple incisional biopsies from involved sites can be taken to effectively 'field map' the histopathological features throughout the oropharynx [6].

We have previously reported the results of examination under anaesthesia and field mapping biopsies for 16 consecutive multiple lesion patients. We found that lesions presenting at the faucial pillars, floor of mouth and ventral tongue were more likely to appear as non-homogeneous leukoplakias or erythroplakias and to exhibit the most severe grades of dysplasia. Mapping the severest dysplastic changes in this way subsequently facilitated targeted laser surgery to specifically excise these areas [6]. Whilst the details of precancer management will be discussed in detail in Chapter 7, we recommend the 'field mapping' technique as an effective tool in the initial identification and subsequent treatment of the most significantly disordered mucosal tissue in multiple lesion patients.

It has been estimated that overall up to 15% of the general population may display some form of mucosal abnormality, the vast majority of which are usually benign conditions. Unfortunately, clinical examination alone cannot discriminate between innocent lesions and potentially malignant ones. Similarly, normal-looking oral mucosa may also harbour molecular abnormalities or even frank histopathological change commensurate with precancer diagnosis in 'at-risk' patients [7].

As clinical examination alone is unlikely to provide improved diagnostic accuracy, it remains important to try to develop diagnostic adjuncts to identify potentially malignant mucosal disease at the earliest possible stage. This has led to the development of newer techniques to characterise precancer change in oral mucosa not visible to the naked eye. Whilst none of these are likely to be used without, nor indeed to replace, visual examination they have been developed to help clinicians in the diagnostic process [2,8]. A list of proposed diagnostic aids for the detection of oral precancer is summarised in Box 5.2, and we will discuss a number of them in this chapter. It is most probably within specialist hospital clinics that such adjunctive technologies will ultimately prove most beneficial, however, because their use in the primary care setting as relatively unfocused screening tools cannot really be recommended.

Box 5.2 Diagnostic aids for clinical detection of oral precancer.

Vital tissue staining
- Toluidine blue

- Lugol's iodine

- 5-aminolevulenic acid

Light-based detection
- Chemiluminescence

- Tissue fluorescence imaging

- Tissue fluorescence spectroscopy

Optical visualisation
- Microcytoscopy

- Optical coherence tomography

Exfoliative cytology
- Brush biopsy and liquid-based cytology

Salivary analysis
- Saliva composition

- Shed oral epithelial cells

In general, a diagnostic adjunct may be used to help identify either the presence of abnormal mucosa in the oral cavity or to determine the risk of malignant transformation in a previously recognised oral lesion. It is likely that in clinical practice, however, there will be a significant overlap between these two objectives.

Diagnostic aids in precancer diagnosis

Vital tissue staining

Vital tissue-staining techniques are based upon the principal that neoplastic and dysplastic tissue may preferentially take up an applied chemical dye. This results in staining and thus identification of abnormal mucosa compared with adjacent normal tissue. Clinical trials to assess the usefulness of such techniques in practice, however, have shown varying results.

One of the most widely studied agents is *toluidine blue* (or tolonium chloride), which is a vital tissue stain that has been used for many years to assist in the detection of mucosal lesions of the cervix and in the oral cavity. It is a metachromatic dye that binds preferentially to rapidly proliferating epithelium, such as that seen in inflammatory, regenerative and neoplastic or dysplastic tissue. It is believed to stain nucleic acids, leading to a retained blue discolouration of abnormal mucosa.

In the oral cavity, patients first undertake a pre-stain oral rinse with 1% acetic acid solution and then gargle with the toluidine blue solution followed by a post-stain rinse of acetic acid. Any persistent blue stain seen on the mucosa is regarded as a positive result, which should either be biopsied then and there, or reviewed again in 14 days time, re-stained and biopsied if persistent.

Whilst not the subject of any significant randomised controlled trials, numerous observational studies have suggested that toluidine blue may have a potential role as a diagnostic aid. Unfortunately, the methodologies of these reported studies vary considerably, as do results for both sensitivity and specificity and very few investigations have compared staining results with a definitive histopathological diagnosis [2].

In general toluidine blue appears to be good at detecting squamous carcinoma, but is only positive in about 50% of oral dysplasia cases. The stain has been shown, however, to preferentially highlight lesions with severe degrees of dysplasia, those with distorted molecular patterns and those with poor clinical outcome or increased risk of progression to malignancy in high-risk populations [2].

It appears, therefore, that whilst toluidine blue may be reliable at detecting established carcinomas or lesions exhibiting severe dysplasia it is less effective in detecting early precancer change. Similarly, there does not appear to be any really significant evidence that toluidine blue can either identify or predict the risk of progression or malignant transformation of mucosal abnormalities that have not already been seen by naked eye examination, which is really the prime objective of a truly useful diagnostic adjunct. Unfortunately, toluidine blue will in addition frequently stain common benign, inflammatory or ulcerative lesions and the stain may also be retained on tongue dorsum crevices, dental plaque deposits and gingiva. This may give rise to substantial confusion in interpreting results, especially in relation to equivocal or pale-staining lesions [2].

These factors, together with the lack of any scientific evidence that toluidine blue is effective as a screening technique in primary care and its somewhat time-consuming method of application have effectively limited its widespread use in clinical practice. And interestingly, in a recent study of toluidine blue use in a large population of nearly 8000 Taiwanese patients in a community screening programme, there was little evidence of any significant advantage when compared with simple visual examination alone [9].

An alternative vital dye technique utilises *Lugol's iodine*, a solution of elemental iodine and potassium iodide in water, that stains the glycogen of normal oral mucosa brown and exposes dysplastic tissue as pale. The same limitations apply to this staining technique as to the use of toluidine blue, however, with the additional disadvantage of its use being restricted to non-keratinised mucosa only [10].

Other workers have reported on the use of haematoporphyrin derivatives, such as *5-aminolevulenic acid*, which may similarly be retained in dysplastic tissue and then visualised by subsequent fluorescence imaging. Once again such techniques are somewhat limited in both effectiveness and applicability.

Overall, it is probably true to say that whilst vital staining may well have some value as an adjunctive aid in specialist dysplasia clinics, especially in the assessment of patients presenting with widespread or multifocal disease, there is currently no evidence to support its efficacy in routine clinical practice or as a primary care screening tool [2,8,9].

Light-based detection systems

Light-based detection systems have developed in recent years as minimally invasive diagnostic visualisation aids to facilitate accurate localisation of dysplastic or neoplastic mucosa. This helps direct biopsies to the most appropriate site thereby reducing diagnostic or treatment delays. In oral oncology practice, the properties of tissue reflectance and narrow emission tissue fluorescence provide the basis for most currently available light-based detection systems [2,8].

Tissue reflectance   Tissue reflectance, for use in oral cancer and precancer identification, was developed following successful use in the uterine cervix. Tissue reflectance units for oral oncology currently marketed include ViziLite® (Zila Pharmaceuticals, Phoenix, AZ, USA) and MicroLux/DL® (AdDent Inc., Danbury, CT, USA), both used in conjunction with a 1% acetic acid mouth rinse solution followed by direct visual examination of the oral cavity using a blue-white light source. This is thus referred to as chemiluminescent illumination.

Acetic acid removes cellular debris and probably dehydrates cells, thus facilitating easier visualisation of the cell nuclei. Dysplastic epithelial cells displaying increased nuclear to cytoplasmic ratios reflect diffuse, low-level chemiluminescent light appearing 'aceto-white' against a bluish normal mucosa background. Toluidine blue solution may be used in addition to mark out the 'aceto-white' lesions for biopsy once the light source is removed (ViziLite Plus®).

Unfortunately, chemiluminescent systems have not, to date, shown significant advantages over clinical examination alone. Whilst chemiluminescence may enhance the visibility of clinically identifiable lesions by improving sharpness and brightness, this hardly justifies the additional costs. Similarly, a number of studies have confirmed that they fail to identify clinically undetectable lesions, they have no predictive value in determining individual lesion behaviour, do not discriminate well between inflammatory, traumatic or potentially malignant lesions, and the presence of distracting visual highlights may actually impair rather than enhance oral examination.

There is thus currently no evidence to recommend chemiluminescence for the detection of occult oral dysplasia and oral squamous carcinoma. The real value of an effective adjunctive diagnostic test, of course, is the ability to identify dysplasia or early squamous cell carcinoma before it becomes clinically apparent.

Narrow emission tissue fluorescence Autofluorescence of tissue under high-intensity light excitation is produced by endogenous fluorophores such as tissue matrix molecules or intracellular collagens, elastins and keratins. In diseased tissue, increased cellular DNA, increasing epithelial thickness, altered collagen content and increased vascularity alter the concentration of fluorophores. This effectively changes the pattern of light scattering and absorption within the tissue thus attenuating excitation and producing colour changes that can be visualised [2,8,11].

The VELscope® (Visually Enhanced Lesion Scope, LED Dental Inc., White Rock, British Columbia, Canada) is a portable hand-held device that allows direct visualisation of the oral cavity. It was developed by LED Medical Diagnostics Inc. in collaboration with the British Columbia Cancer Agency. Figure 5.11A shows the VELscope instrument, which is only a little larger than a conventional laptop personal computer, whilst in Figure 5.11B the hand-held scope is being used for

(A)

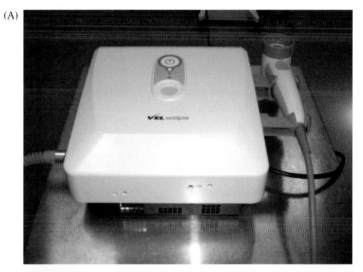

(B)

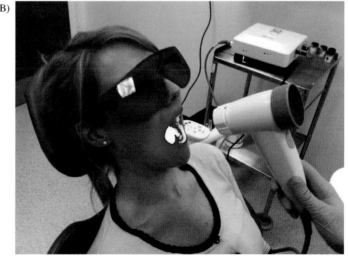

Figure 5.11 (A) The VELscope is just larger than a laptop PC and is easily accommodated in both out-patient clinics and operating theatres. (B) The VELscope being used in a clinic during an oral mucosal examination.

(A)   (B)

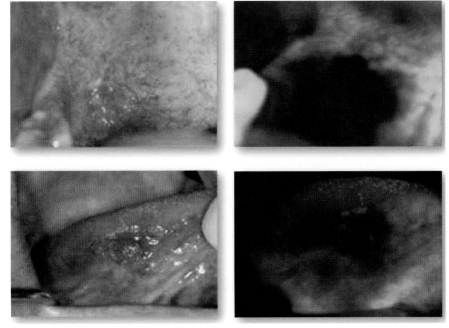

Figure 5.12 (A) Clinical appearance of
dysplastic mucosal lesions arising in the
posterior floor of mouth and ventrolateral
tongue and (B) the resultant dark
appearance seen upon VELscope
examination compared with the normal
green-white mucosal background. (Images
courtesy of VELscope, LED Dental Inc.)

oral examination in the out-patient clinic. Under an intense, 400–460 nm blue
excitation light, normal mucosa emits a pale green autofluorescence when viewed
through the handpiece filter, whilst carcinoma or dysplastic tissue appears dark as
a result of decreased normal autofluorescence (Figure 5.12).

A significant practical advantage of this technique is the portability of the
instrument, which can be used in clinics or operating theatre environments.
The fact that neither acetic acid nor toluidine blue mucosal treatments or
mouthwashes are required prior to examination by VELscope is also useful.

No randomised controlled clinical trials have yet been carried out to compare
this device with other diagnostic methods, but a number of preliminary reports
suggest that the VELscope is capable of identifying dysplastic tissue not seen on
conventional visual examination. Comparing VELscope examination with
histopathological biopsy data has shown 98% sensitivity and 100% specificity
for discriminating dysplasia and carcinoma from normal oral mucosa.

Goodson et al. used the VELscope to examine 100 patients with dysplastic
oral lesions and found the technique helpful in identifying abnormal sites for
mucosal biopsy and reasonably accurate in predicting dysplasia at those
sites [12]. However, the VELscope proved less reliable during the examination
of follow-up patients where dark changes consequent upon stromal neovascu-
larisation seen at previous biopsy or laser surgery scar sites could confuse the
autofluorescence imaging.

Overall, however, we feel the VELscope shows promise as a diagnostic tool in
precancer diagnosis and it is now routinely used in our clinical practice. Its
particular value is that it is a highly portable instrument, is quick and easy to use
and is very acceptable to patients. Multicentre, prospective, randomised clinical
trials are now indicated to determine its true efficacy as a reliable adjunct in the
diagnosis of potentially malignant disorders.

Tissue fluorescence spectroscopy   This is a relatively new technique in which a
small optical fibre producing different excitation wavelengths is applied to the
oral mucosa. The resultant spectra of reflected tissue fluorescence is then analysed

in an objective manner by computer. The main disadvantage is that the probe size limits its use to small, localised lesions and, once again, is only really useful once an abnormal lesion has been found on prior visual examination [8,13].

Brush biopsy and exfoliative cytology

Exfoliative cytology is essentially the analysis and interpretation of the characteristics of cells shed from mucosal surfaces. Oral exfoliative cytology largely developed following techniques used in cytology of the uterine cervix but has never really achieved the same successful application in oral diagnosis and is not in widespread clinical use, still remaining largely a research tool. Difficulties in the development of oral cytology are mainly due to problems in acquiring cytology specimens of significant diagnostic quality from appropriate locations to provide accurate representation of the dysplastic nature of lesions from which they were obtained.

Whilst a variety of instruments, including cotton applicator sticks, gel and cellulose foam, wooden or metal spatulas have been used to collect cells, all techniques have had difficulty in obtaining cells from the basal layer of oral epithelium. Most dysplastic changes arise in the basal epithelial layers and cells often lose their dysplastic characteristics as they mature, travelling from basal to superficial layers, with nuclei become less visible and keratinisation making accurate grading of dysplasia difficult.

A system of obtaining exfoliated cells by cell collection devices known as cytobrushes, such as the OralCDx® brush (Oral CDx Laboratories Inc., Suffern, NY, USA), has been devised to increase basal cell yield. This is achieved through full-thickness sampling of stratified epithelium, although cell clumping, epithelial fragmentation and lack of epithelial structural hierarchy seen on glass slide microscopy limit its usefulness compared with histopathological examination. It is also best considered as a diagnostic 'step' rather than a definitive diagnostic test as an incisional biopsy must follow an abnormal result; it may even be superfluous when clinical appearances are suspicious, dictating histopathological assessment [8].

More recently the Orcellex® brush (Rovers Medical Devices B.V., the Netherlands) [14], a novel cytobrush using 'thin hair technology', has been developed. The specially designed brush head, which comprises five segments of high-density fibres designed for optimal cell collection, is shown in Figure 5.13.

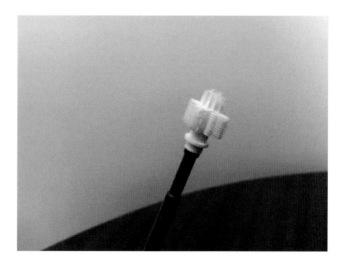

Figure 5.13 Close-up view of the Orcellex brush head, which comprises five segments of high-density fibres that allow optimal collection, storage and release of cell material.

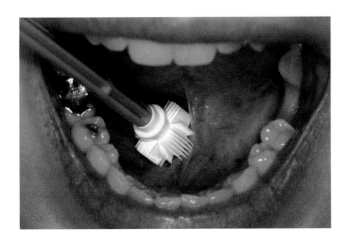

Figure 5.14 Orcellex brush applied to the floor of mouth mucosa to harvest epithelial cells for cytology. The brush is placed firmly against the mucosa and rotated ten times.

Adequate cellular samples, containing representative cells from all oral epithelial layers, can be obtained by rotating the brush ten times against the oral mucosa. The use of the brush in harvesting cells from floor of mouth tissue is illustrated in Figure 5.14.

Liquid-based cytology, rather than conventional glass slide smears, has been evaluated for use with the Orcellex brush biopsy. This appears to improve cell distribution, to reduce cell clumping and to assist in production of thin layer preparations that can be used for accurate cytological evaluation and subsequent biomarker profiling [14,15]. Figure 5.15 shows the typical appearance of a liquid based cytology preparation following an oral brush biopsy

As premalignant changes occur at the molecular level before they are seen microscopically or clinically, biomolecular assessment of exfoliated cells together with DNA, RNA and microRNA analyses may all contribute to a minimally invasive genetic screening approach for both the detection and monitoring of oral precancer, especially following interventional treatment [16].

In a small study of 30 consecutive new patients presenting with oral potentially malignant lesions, we found the Orcellex brush to be reliable in identifying aytpia and dyskaryosis in exfoliated cell samples, to accurately correspond to subsequent histopathological diagnoses in the majority of cases and, importantly, to be very acceptable to patients as a non-invasive and reasonably comfortable investigation [17,18].

Indeed, if the accuracy of brush cytology can be confirmed to be as good as histopathological examination, it may well have a significant clinical use. This would be particularly in the assessment of large mucosal abnormalities, multiple or persistent lesions, and for non-compliant or irregular clinic attenders where repeat biopsies may be inconvenient, uncomfortable or impractical for patients. It remains to be seen, however, whether exfoliative cytology will truly develop from a primarily research methodology into a universally applicable clinical diagnostic tool. An important disadvantage of exfoliative epithelial cell examination remains the inability to assess epithelial structural hierarchy and the lack of visualisation of epithelial–connective tissue interactions which are only facilitated by conventional biopsy techniques. Indeed, many authors consider brush biopsy will only ever be likely to serve as an intermediate diagnostic procedure, perhaps primarily to investigate lesions where there is a low level of clinical suspicion, because most clinicians faced with uncertainty over a mucosal lesion would, and indeed probably should, undertake a biopsy for histopathological examination [2,13].

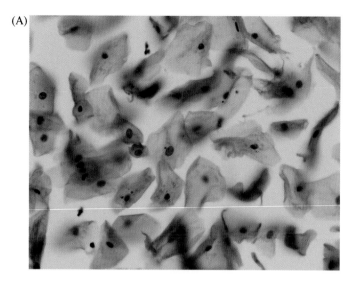

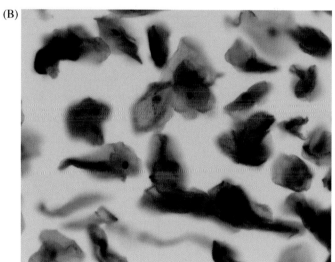

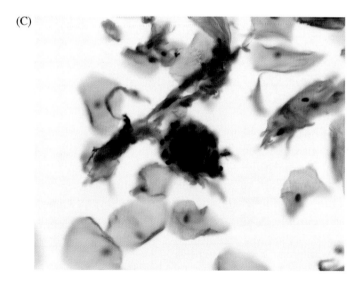

Figure 5.15 Brush biopsy in conjunction with liquid-based cytology produces samples with up to 50 000 epithelial cells per slide, allowing identification of basal and parabasal cells (A), intermediate layer cells (B) and superficial cells (C) as well as distinguishing individual cell atypia and dyskaryosis.

Clinical diagnosis in practice

A truly comprehensive clinical diagnosis of oral precancer disease requires more than simply ascribing terms and nomenclature to a particular oral lesion, although unfortunately this is often all that is currently achievable. A thorough diagnosis should, ideally, identify and categorise the patient and their lesion into either a 'high-risk' or 'low-risk' category for disease progression and malignant transformation, describe both the site and extent of oral mucosa involved and detail the provisional incisional biopsy histopathology report. Assessment of the potential for field change and multiple lesion disease should also be carried out and documented.

In this way, we should be trying to achieve individual patient disease profiling, which should lead to rationalisation of both diagnostic and clinical management protocols.

Summary

In order to improve patient morbidity and mortality from oral cancer, early detection and treatment of potentially malignant disease remains essential. Thorough and methodical visual examination of the oral mucosa by an experienced clinician, using sound clinical judgement, supplemented by targeted incisional biopsy for histopathological classification, remains the 'gold standard' for diagnosis. It is recommended that clinicians should remain alert for signs of potentially malignant lesions and early signs of cancer in all patients when performing routine oral and dental examinations. This is especially so for patients who use tobacco and consume alcohol [19].

Unfortunately, potentially malignant disorders demonstrate a considerable heterogeneity in clinical presentation and even with a high index of suspicion many lesions may be missed or mistaken for benign conditions.

In recent years there has been a rapid development of diagnostic aids as potential screening or case finding tools but none have been scientifically validated. Clinical reporting of their use is highly anecdotal and there is no strong evidence to support the application of any one particular technique.

Whilst computer analysis of cytology specimens, biomolecular categorisation of shed epithelial cells in saliva, and techniques based upon confocal microscopy, optical coherence microscopy and tomography offer future promise, it remains unlikely that any single technique will ultimately prove superior to clinical examination [20]. Furthermore, we must recognise the current limitations of conventional diagnostic techniques. In the future, molecular and genetic profiling of potentially malignant tissue will undoubtedly supplement and may ultimately exceed existing clinical and histopathological assessments [14,21]. We will return to a more detailed discussion of some of these future technologies in Chapter 10.

References

1. Kujan O, Glenny A-M, Duxbury J, Thakker N, Sloan P. Evaluation of screening strategies for improving oral cancer mortality: a Cochrane systematic review. *J Dent Educ* 2005; 69: 255–265.

2. Lingen MW, Kalmar JR, Karrison T, Speight PM. Critical evaluation of diagnostic aids for the detection of oral cancer. *Oral Oncol* 2008; 44: 10–22.

3. Brocklehurst PR, Baker SR, Speight PM. A qualitative study examining the experience of primary care dentists in the detection and management of potentially malignant lesions. 1. Factors influencing detection and the decision to refer. *Br Dent J* 2010; 208: E3.

4. McGurk M, Scott SE. The reality of identifying early oral cancer in the general dental practice. *Br Dent J* 2010; 208: 347–351.

5. Thomson PJ, Wylie J. Interventional laser surgery: an effective surgical and diagnostic tool in oral precancer management. *Int J Oral Maxillofac Surg* 2002; 31: 145–153.

6. Thomson PJ, Hamadah O. Cancerisation within the oral cavity: the use of 'field mapping biopsies' in clinical management. *Oral Oncol* 2007; 43: 20–26.

7. Thomson PJ. Field change and oral cancer: new evidence for widespread carcinogenesis? *Int J Oral Maxillofac Surgery* 2002; 31: 262–266.

8. Fedele S. Diagnostic aids in the screening of oral cancer. *Head Neck Oncol* 2009; 1: 5.

9. Su WW, Yen AM, Chiu SY, Chen TH. A community-based RCT for oral cancer screening with toluidine blue. *J Dent Res* 2010; 89: 933–937.

10. Petruzzi M, Lucchese A, Baldoni E, Grassi FR, Serpico R. Use of Lugol's iodine in oral cancer diagnosis: an overview. *Oral Oncol* 2010; 46: 811–813.

11. Vigneswaran N, Koh S, Gillenwater A. Incidental detection of an occult oral malignancy with autofluorescence imaging: a case report. *Head Neck Oncol* 2009; 1: 37.

12. Goodson ML, Diajil A, Sloan P, Thomson PJ. VELscope: an effective tool for diagnosis and follow up of oral precancer patients. *Eur Arch Otorhinolaryngol* 2010; 267 (Suppl 1): S72.

13. Leston JS, Dios PD. Diagnostic clinical aids in oral cancer. *Oral Oncol* 2010; 46: 418–422.

14. Sloan P. Oral cancer screening. *Cytopathology* 2007; 18 (Suppl 1): 12.

15. Epstein JB, Zhang L, Rosin M. Advances in the diagnosis of oral premalignant and malignant lesions. *J Can Dent Assoc* 2002; 68: 617–621.

16. Bremmer JF, Graveland AP, Brink A. et al. Screening for oral precancer with noninvasive genetic technology. *Cancer Prev Res* 2009; 2: 128–133.

17. Thomson PJ, Goodson ML, Wadhera V, Johnson S, Sloan P. Brush cytology: preliminary results using the 'Orcellex' brush. *15th International Congress on Oral Pathology and Medicine Abstract Book*, 2010: 138.

18. Goodson ML, Wadhera V, Johnson S, Thomson PJ, Sloan P. Patient satisfaction with the 'Orcellex' brush. *15th International Congress on Oral Pathology and Medicine Abstract Book*, 2010: 137.

19. Richards D. Clinical recommendations for oral cancer screening. *Evidence-Based Dent* 2010; 11: 101–102.

20. Gillenwater A, Papadimitrakopoulou V, Richards-Kortum R. Oral premalignancy: new methods of detection and treatment. *Curr Oncol Rep* 2006; 8: 146–154.

21. Kao S-Y, Chu Y-W, Chen Y-W, Chang K-W, Liu T-Y. Detection and screening of oral cancer and pre-cancerous lesions. *J Chin Med Assoc* 2009; 72: 227–233.

6 Pathological Aspects of Oral Precancer

Philip Sloan

Oral Precancer: Diagnosis and Management of Potentially Malignant Disorders, First Edition. Edited by Peter Thomson.
© 2012 John Wiley & Sons, Ltd. Published 2012 by John Wiley & Sons, Ltd.

Introduction

Oral epithelial dysplasia is the histopathological term used to describe a spectrum of tissue dysmaturation and disorganisation changes, involving both architectural disturbance and cytological atypia, seen in biopsy specimens taken from oral potentially malignant lesions. The presence of such dysplastic regions within oral epithelium is thought to be associated with an enhanced possibility of malignant transformation, with the most severe dysplasias probably at greatest risk.

The identification and subsequent grading of the severity of dysplastic change is thus fundamental to oral precancer diagnosis and its subsequent management. The relationship and communication between the clinician in the dysplasia clinic and the pathologist in the laboratory, therefore, is absolutely central to accurate diagnosis, clinical decision making, treatment planning and ultimately, of course, the overall welfare of oral potentially malignant disorder patients.

Interpreting the significance of clinically observed oral mucosal lesions requires tissue samples to be obtained by biopsy and transported to the laboratory for specialised histopathological assessment and diagnosis. Although molecular biology is being increasingly used in oncology research, traditional light microscopic assessment of formalin-fixed tissue remains the cornerstone of diagnostic pathology and is likely to remain so for many years to come.

In this chapter we will explore the fundamental principles of pathological science as applied to the diagnosis and management of oral precancer.

Biopsy techniques

Accurate pathological diagnosis is reliant on appropriate sampling of the oral potentially malignant lesion. In Chapter 5, we discussed the diagnostic process for potentially malignant disorders and emphasised the fundamental importance of biopsy. It is vital that the clinician selects the most appropriate sites for biopsy and, on occasion, multiple samples may be required to map widespread field change.

Except for very small lesions, it is usual to perform incisional biopsies first to obtain a tissue diagnosis. It is well recognised that invasive carcinoma may be diagnosed in unexpected situations; examples include flat white or red mucosal patches and erythematous gingival lesions. Consequently biopsy of any suspicious, non-healing or unexplained oral lesions is mandatory.

Incisional biopsies of potentially malignant lesions must be adequate in size and of sufficient depth to include the reticular lamina propria. Achieving sufficient depth can be a problem with thick keratinising lesions. Elliptical scalpel biopsies have been used for many years but there is an increasing preference for the punch biopsy [1]. Punch biopsy instruments are available in a range of diameters up to 10 mm. Before taking the biopsy, local analgesia should be achieved by injection around (but not directly into) the mucosal area to be sampled. After making a circular incision the punch biopsy can be released with minimal trauma using scissors.

The biopsy should be placed immediately into at least ten times its volume of fixative. Normally the laboratory providing the diagnostic service will provide pre-filled biopsy containers with advice on labelling, transporting to the laboratory and other issues to ensure an effective and safe service.

From the point of view of the pathologist, mucosal punch biopsies offer many advantages. Standard operating procedures can be devised to ensure a consistent approach in the pathology laboratory to specimen trimming, biopsy orientation, embedding and sectioning with preparation of appropriate levels. A more rapid turnaround time is facilitated and problems with interpretation of poorly orientated biopsies can be minimised.

In oral potentially malignant lesions the interface between the oral epithelium and lamina propria can be complex, particularly in thick lesions. Adverse orientation of sections can exaggerate the complex architecture and lead to difficulties in recognising whether invasion is present or not. Punch biopsies have been reported to cause less morbidity than scalpel biopsies and can be closed with a single suture or left to heal by primary intention. In a volunteer study to assess tolerance of 3 mm buccal punch biopsies, all subjects stated that they would be willing to undergo a subsequent biopsy procedure [2].

A limitation of even multiple punch biopsy evaluation is sampling. One powerful argument favouring laser excision of oral potentially malignant lesions is that the entire clinical lesion can be sampled. Sometimes this leads to a diagnosis of invasive carcinoma that was not suspected clinically. Standard operating procedures for trimming laser excisions should be used in the pathology laboratory. The specimen should be accompanied by a diagram or photograph and orientation sutures can be inserted. Figure 6.1 demonstrates a laser excision specimen immediately following surgery with orientation sutures in situ to distinguish the anterior and lateral excision margins. Mucosal margins can also be inked. Serial blocking techniques are most effective and good clinical correlation is needed to ensure clarity of diagnosis in relation to margin status.

A large body of literature has accumulated describing molecular alterations in pathways that control cellular signalling, cytoskeleton development, cell cycles, apoptosis, genomic stability and angiogenesis, amongst others. Many of these studies suffer from cross-sectional design, a relatively small sample size

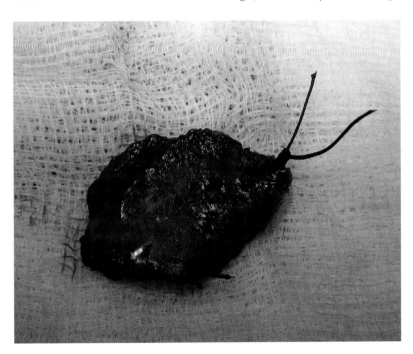

Figure 6.1 Laser excision specimen showing orientation sutures at the anterior and lateral excision margins.

and a lack of consistent diagnostic criteria. No biomarkers are currently used in routine practice for the evaluation of oral potentially malignant disorders. A promising approach is combined analysis, for example the detection of aneuploidy with other biomarkers in sections or even single cells [3,4].

Exfoliative oral cytology has an increasing role for the evaluation of oral potentially malignant lesions [4] and in recognising dysplasia in suspicious oral lesions with both high sensitivity and specificity [5,6]. The use of auxiliary methods such as DNA image cytometry, AgNOR analysis and cell cycle immunohistochemistry can increase accuracy even further [5,7]. A biopsy must be performed, however, whenever dysplasia is detected, not only because the architecture needs to be considered when grading lesions but also because invasion cannot be reliably assessed by exfoliative cytology alone. Dysplasia can be assessed cytologically using direct smears or by liquid-based cytology methods.

The recognised cytological features of oral dysplasia are:

- Nuclear hyperchromasia.

- Increased nuclear to cytoplasmic ratio.

- Anisonucleosis and nuclear pleomorphism.

- Irregularities of nuclear membrane.

- Nuclear crowding.

- Nuclear moulding, clumping and irregular distribution of chromatin.

Cytological diagnosis is skill dependent and the cytopathologist must be able to recognise regenerating oral epithelial cells, which often form aggregates of immature keratinocytes. These cells may exhibit an increased nuclear to cytoplasmic ratio and sometimes possess prominent nucleoli, but may show no other nuclear abnormalities. Radiation- and chemoradiation-induced changes including micronucleation must be considered when cytology is performed in the immediate post-irradiation setting [4,8].

Role of the pathologist

In the absence of accurate predictive biomarkers, histological examination of biopsies is the current standard for planning the management of oral potentially malignant lesions. A number of grading systems for evaluation of dysplasia have been proposed and are discussed in the next section. Unfortunately, a number of studies have demonstrated that agreement amongst even specialist oral and maxillofacial pathologists is only fair, with kappa values typically ranging between 0.5 and 0.6.

Binary grading systems that classify lesions into 'low grade' and 'high grade' show improved utility in terms of predictive value and inter-observer agreement [9]. An agreement level of around 80% was reached when pathologists were asked to discriminate between dysplasia (of any grade) and cases without dysplasia [10]. Group training relating to criteria for defining the features of dysplasia appears to increase reliability. Non-specialist pathologists tend to downgrade oral dysplasia compared to specialist oral and maxillofacial pathologists [9]. It is interesting that even when pathologists agree on the grade they may be basing their judgement on differing features [11].

Factors such as the presence or absence of lichenoid inflammation, clinical history (smoking and alcohol use) and lesion site have been reported to consistently influence dysplasia grading [12]. It is regrettable that clinical treatment planning has to be performed on the basis of pathology reports that show such poor reliability. Biomarkers are needed that have the power to predict biological behaviour but as yet no markers have proved to be sufficiently robust for clinical application. Clinical correlation can help, and close involvement of the pathologist with the clinical team is facilitated by specialist pathology reporting. Consensus reporting of oral dysplasia by a team of specialist pathologists also helps to improve reporting accuracy and over time develops greater consistency.

A dedicated laboratory team experienced in orientating mucosal specimens correctly and agreed protocols defining the number of levels prepared are also important in providing a high-quality service. Regular review (audit) and the monitoring of clinical outcomes in a comprehensive database that includes pathological findings are useful tools for developing optimal management protocols.

The relative rarity and huge variability of oral potentially malignant lesions makes it difficult to undertake randomised controlled trials. Prolonged follow-up times, which are needed for potential lesions to reach malignant transformation, also hamper such trials. The accrual of a biobank of samples of oral potentially malignant lesions accompanied by clinical data, including outcomes, is necessary for future biomarker evaluation. Input from specialist pathologists is therefore vital not only for the provision of day to day reporting services but also to the development of long-term goals.

Histopathological features of oral potentially malignant disorders

The concept that squamous carcinoma has a prolonged preinvasive phase that offers the opportunity for therapeutic intervention was first recognised in the cervix. Indeed, early descriptions of the cytological and architectural histological features of oral precancerous lesions largely evolved from previous accounts of their cervical counterparts. Unfortunately, the epithelium of the uterine cervix is dissimilar in many ways to the oral mucosa, which is itself heterogeneous in nature, as described in Chapter 2.

The epithelium of the cervix is non-keratinising and varies during reproductive life. Cervical squamous epithelium differentiates by metaplasia from the reserve cell population that normally replenishes the columnar cells of the endocervical canal, and a transitional zone can be recognised histologically. Also in contrast to oral cancer, most cervical cancers are human papillomavirus (HPV) related and this may influence the morphology of cervical intraepithelial neoplasia (CIN) [13].

The CIN system encompasses six stages, from normal through reactive, CIN1, CIN2 and CIN3, to invasion; these can be mapped to the squamous intraepithelial neoplasia (SIN) system (Figure 6.2). These are thought to represent a serial progression but evidence for this is lacking due to the ethics constraints of designing a clinical trial to determine if there is a succession of events. In a widely quoted, extended and unethical clinical trial it was demonstrated that the 30-year cumulative risk of cervical cancer was 0.7% in women with adequately treated CIN, in contrast to 31.3% in those managed only by diagnostic biopsy [14].

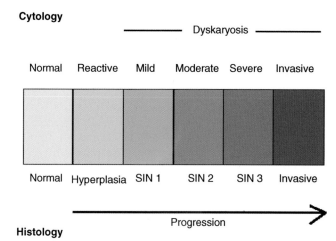

Figure 6.2 The concept of progression, initially proposed in models of cervical intraepithelial neoplasia, has been applied to head and neck grading systems.

Figures for the transformation of oral precancerous lesions are very variable but are generally lower than the malignant transformation rate of at least 30% that is widely accepted for CIN3. Concepts of oral carcinogenesis have been outlined in Chapter 3, whilst Chapter 9 will review malignant transformation of oral potentially malignant disorders.

The current gold standard for diagnosis of oral precancer, which are often described as precursor lesions, is the World Health Organisation(WHO) classification [15]. Building on the famous WHO 'Blue Book' of 1971, the updated classification seeks to harmonise the SIN, WHO and Ljubljana grading systems. The 2005 WHO classification also defines individual cytological and architectural features of dysplasia, and is summarised in Table 6.1. Numerous challenges are set for the pathologist, which include overlap between the described features, the omission of some features such as acantholysis, and the problem of how to weight each dysplastic feature.

A further possible confounding factor is the entity known as proliferative verrucous leukoplakia (PVL), described in a separate chapter in the WHO 2005 classification. This is a distinctive and often multifocal precursor lesion with a very high risk of ultimate transformation. Some authors describe PVL as inevitably transforming, despite having mainly architectural abnormalities with sometimes minimal cytological atypia.

The organisation of pathology services into large diagnostic laboratories with rapid turnaround times and accreditation requirements has resulted in oral biopsies often being reported by non-specialists. Reports are often written with

Architecture	Cytology
Irregular epithelial stratification	Abnormal variation in nuclear size (anisonucleosis)
Loss of polarity of basal cells	Abnormal variation in nuclear shape (nuclear pleomorphism)
Drop-shaped rete ridges	Abnormal variation in cell size (anisocytosis)
Increased number of mitotic figures	Abnormal variation in cell shape (cellular pleomorphism)
Abnormally superficial mitoses	Increased nuclear to cytoplasmic ratio
Premature keratinisation in single cells (dyskeratosis)	Increased nuclear size
Keratin pearls within rete pegs	Atypical mitotic figures
	Increased number and size of nucleoli
	Hyperchromasia

Table 6.1 Features of dysplasia in oral potentially malignant lesions (WHO tumour classification 2005).

minimal clinical information. Consequently, pathologists typically describe the observed features, particularly any epithelial cytological atypia and architectural abnormalities, and then attempt to ascribe a dysplasia grading.

Issues relating to dysplasia grading will be discussed in the next section. However it is not clear from the current WHO 2005 classification whether pathologists should 'sign out' a diagnosis of PVL where possible or simply give a histological grading on all submitted suspicious lesions. Several studies have shown poor inter-observer agreement between even specialist oral pathologists on dysplasia grading and these issues will be explored in more detail in the next section [9,10,12].

Grading of dysplasia

World health organisation system

The WHO first defined an oral premalignant lesion as 'a morphologically altered tissue in which oral cancer was more likely to occur than in its apparently normal counterpart' in 1973. Under this early WHO classification, atypical epithelium was divided into two pathological entities, one with progression to squamous cell carcinoma and the other remaining stable or regressing. Epithelial dysplasia, which was divided into mild, moderate or severe categories, was recognised to occur in both types of lesion. With time, an increasing degree of dysplasia was assumed to represent progression. This view of a progression model has remained unchanged from the first edition of the WHO 'Blue Book' in 1971 to the latest edition in 2005, which incorporates both pathology and genetics [15].

Dysplasia in oral mucosa is characterised by both cellular and architectural atypia. Individual features of dysplasia are recognised by the pathologist and listed, and lesions are then graded into one of four different categories: mild, moderate or severe dysplasia, or carcinoma in situ (CIS). The latter is considered to be preinvasive malignancy at the extreme end of epithelial dysplasia. Figures 6.3 and 6.4 illustrate the histopathological features of mild dysplasia, whilst Figure 6.5 demonstrates moderately dysplastic epithelium.

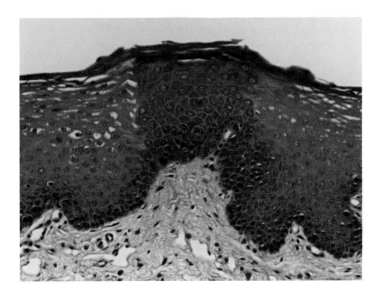

Figure 6.3 Mild epithelial dysplasia. Sharply defined columns of cells possessing more basophilic cytoplasm may represent early genetic stem cell alterations in a proliferation unit.

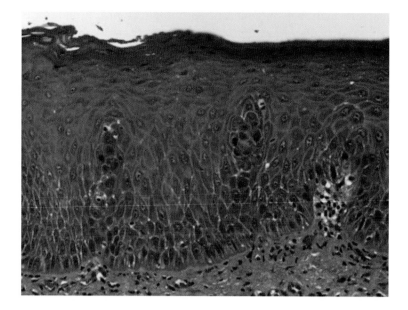

Figure 6.4 Mild epithelial dysplasia in the floor of the mouth. Basal cell hyperplasia and parakeratosis are present.

The current WHO classification provides a table listing 16 recognised features of dysplasia divided into architectural and cytological features. One fundamental problem is that there is no evidence to indicate how individual features should be weighted. Furthermore, many pathologists recognise that acantholysis, which is a loss of cell cohesion, is often observed in oral dysplasia but the feature is not recognised in the WHO classification. Figure 6.6 shows an example of acantholysis in a dysplastic lesion.

Generally, pathologists attempt to grade individual lesions on the basis that the more numerous or more prominent the abnormal factors are perceived to be, the more severe is the grade of dysplasia. It is also necessary to determine whether the features are limited to the lower third of the epithelium (mild dysplasia), extend to two-thirds of the epithelium (moderate dysplasia) or involve more than two-thirds (severe dysplasia). Figure 6.7 is an example of severe epithelial dysplasia. The terms 'full thickness' or 'almost full thickness' architectural abnormalities are recommended for use in applying the diagnosis of CIS (Figure 6.8).

Figure 6.9 shows the histopathological features of PVL, whilst Figure 6.10 illustrates the development of squamous cell carcinoma, which is known to be a high-risk occurrence, arising from a background of PVL.

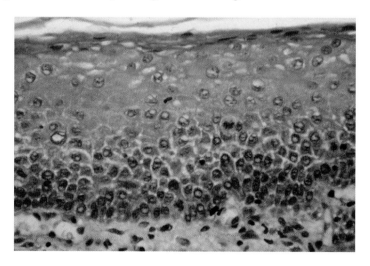

Figure 6.5 Moderate dysplasia, as shown in an incisional biopsy from a floor of mouth erythroleukoplakia lesion.

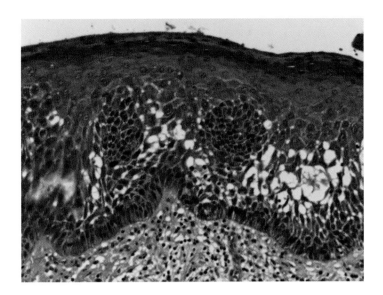

Figure 6.6 Acantholysis is often seen in oral dysplasia, although it is not a recognised feature in the WHO classification of 2005.

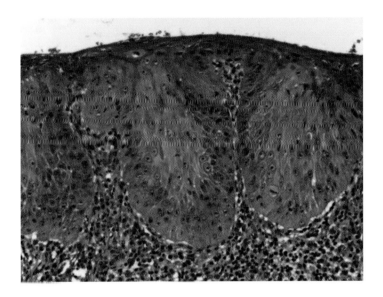

Figure 6.7 Severe epithelial dysplasia with a thin parakeratin layer on the surface; this can be considered as 'differentiated carcinoma in situ'. The SIN 3 category unifies severe dysplasia and carcinoma in situ.

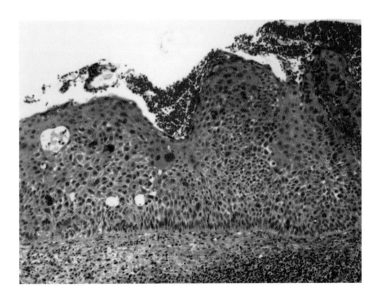

Figure 6.8 Carcinoma in situ in the buccal mucosa. Full thickness cytological atypia is present.

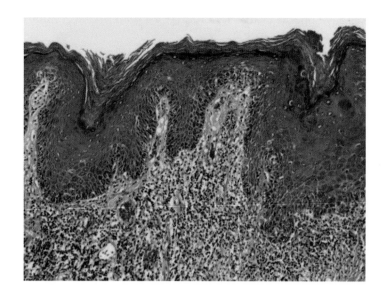

Figure 6.9 Biopsy from a patient with a clinical diagnosis of proliferative verrucous leukoplakia. The patient had extensive white plaques for years. Earlier biopsies showed only lichenoid mucositis, but this biopsy revealed architectural and cytological atypia in the buccal mucosa.

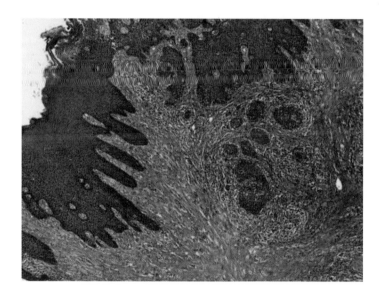

Figure 6.10 Two years after a buccal biopsy was taken the patient developed a thickened lesion in the tongue (same patient as shown in Figure 6.7). The biopsy showed invasive carcinoma arising in a background of proliferative verrucous leukoplakia.

The WHO system is thus complex and may underpin the reported subjectivity of precancer diagnosis [16]. Indeed, many studies have demonstrated marked inter- and intra-observer variability of the grading system [9–12]. To achieve more objective reporting, a greater understanding and the identification of distinct criteria for grading dysplasia are required, and perhaps a less complex system. To this end, a novel binary grading system designed to simplify the WHO classification and to increase reproducibility of diagnosis has been proposed. This system distinguishes 'high-grade' lesions, which tend to be the more severe dysplasias, from 'low-grade' or less severe ones [9,16].

Squamous intraepithelial neoplasia system

The formulation of the SIN system was based on a view that the biology of the squamous mucosa lining the upper aerodigestive tract differs from that of the uterine cervix. Superficial maturation may be seen in association with high-grade cytological atypia in the lower one-third or two-thirds of the upper aerodigestive tract lining squamous epithelium. Therefore application of the criteria used in the WHO system, itself derived from the CIN system, results in underassessment of grade.

While surface keratinisation is uncommon in dysplasia of the uterine cervix it is frequently seen in dysplastic lesions of the upper aerodigestive tract. The advantage of the SIN system is that it recognises 'keratinising dysplasia', which is a term defining severe cytological atypia in the lower part of the epithelium accompanied by surface keratinisation, as a high-grade lesion with frequent progression and transformation to malignancy [17].

Ljubljana classification

The Ljubljana classification was devised by Kambic and Lenart [18] and has been used most widely for the grading of laryngeal lesions. The criteria for histological grading were refined by the Working Group on Head and Neck Pathology of the European Society of Pathology in 1997 [19].

The Ljubljana system describes four grades: *simple hyperplasia* and *basal/parabasal cell hyperplasia*, which are benign categories with a very low risk of malignant transformation, *atypical hyperplasia*, which has malignant potential, and *carcinoma in situ*, which is considered to be a malignant lesion.

The main features that differentiate the Ljubljana grading system from other classifications are the fundamental distinctions between mainly benign (squamous hyperplasia and basal/parabasal hyperplasia) and potentially malignant (atypical hyperplasia) lesions, and the definite separation of CIS from atypical hyperplasia. These two latter entities differ in both morphology and their pattern of progression to invasive carcinoma.

Although the Ljubljana grading system is widely accepted as a useful classification in relation to laryngeal pathology, there is little evidence in the literature relating to its use in the oral mucosa.

Combining the grading systems

Recently, a scheme has been proposed that utilises a binary system that unites the SIN classification and the Ljubljana classification (Table 6.2) [17]. In practice a proportion of potentially malignant lesions are self-limiting and reversible, whilst others remain stable, and some transform to squamous cell carcinoma despite careful follow up and interventions.

Although both classifications can be combined, and there is some limited evidence for the utility of a binary system for grading oral lesions, further work to validate their use in oral mucosa is required. Ideally the WHO, SIN and Ljubljana classifications should be harmonised.

It is of interest to note that the Japanese Society of Oral Pathology has formulated guidelines that build on the WHO classification but incorporate some concepts similar to those proposed by the authors of the SIN classification [20]. One important feature of the Japanese proposal is that it recognises 'differentiated' CIS as well as conventional 'basaloid' CIS. The former is often reported as 'severe dysplasia amounting to carcinoma in situ', and the recognition that CIS can be keratinising on the surface is a step forward in achieving a better classification.

Classification	Hyperplastic form	Atrophic form
Hyperplasia/keratosis	Thickened, hyperplastic epithelium Rare mitosis confined to suprabasal layer Normal maturation Surface keratinisation common No nuclear pleomorphism	Atrophy Thin mucosa Normal mucosal maturation No nuclear pleomorphism
SIN 1 (low grade)	Epithelial hyperplasia Increased mitoses common (1–2 per HPF) Three or more layers of basal-like cells Minor nuclear pleomorphism	Some proliferation of basal-like cells Increased mitoses (1–2 per HPF) Minor nuclear pleomorphism Surface maturation still evident
SIN 2 (high grade)	Epithelial hyperplasia Mitoses in all layers common, including abnormal forms Marked epithelial maturation abnormalities with immature basal-like cells constituting inner and middle one-third or in combination with premature keratinisation, including presence of pearls Prominent nuclear pleomorphism Increased chromatin staining	Proliferation of basal-like cells involving the full thickness Prominent submucosal changes Numerous mitoses at all levels; may have abnormal mitotic forms Prominent nuclear pleomorphism Little or no evidence of maturation or keratinisation

HPF, high power field.

Table 6.2 The combined squamous intraepithelial neoplasia (SIN) and Ljubljana grading systems.

Limitations in conventional pathological techniques

Conventional histopathological methods of assessing oral potentially malignant lesions are currently the gold standard for diagnosis and management, even though they are subjective, imperfect and cannot reliably predict biological behaviour. As yet no useful biomarkers have translated into routine practice. Clinical factors are an important part of diagnosis and it may be that risk models that integrate pathological findings with clinical factors may translate into practice in the future [21].

A retrospective audit of cases retrieved from databases is a useful exercise for the whole clinical team. In one such local audit, our group identified a cohort of patients with oral cancer from the laboratory pathology database. It was possible to identify those who had had previous biopsies of non-neoplastic oral potentially malignant lesions. Dysplasia had not been identified in a significant proportion of these possible precursor lesions, particularly those in which lichenoid inflammation was present [22].

In an attempt to overcome present limitations of conventional techniques, specialist pathology teams should be developed, working closely with their clinical team. Within specialist pathology teams consensus reporting, training, research, innovation and ongoing audit will ultimately improve diagnostic accuracy and prognostication for oral potentially malignant lesions.

Summary

Epithelial dysplasia is a collective histopathological term used to describe tissue structural changes seen by light microscopy in oral potentially malignant disorders. It is, effectively, the histological marker of precancer and as such its presence and severity may be predictive of an increased risk of squamous cell carcinoma development. There are, unfortunately, no consistently reliable histopathological predictors of clinical behaviour and there may also be considerable intra- and inter-observer variation amongst pathologists in the assessment of both the presence and extent of dysplasia. A number of different grading systems have been proposed and are currently in use to try to standardise histopathological diagnoses. Excellent communication and close working relationships between clinicians and specialist pathologists are essential to optimise clinical management strategies for individual patients. In the next chapter we will consider how, following clinical diagnosis and histopathological assessment, potentially malignant disorder cases may be managed clinically.

References

1. Oliver RJ, Sloan P, Pemberton MN. Oral biopsies: methods and applications *Br Dent J* 2004; 196: 329–333.
2. Camidge DR, Pemberton MN, Growcott JW et al. Assessing proliferation, cell cycle arrest and apoptotic end points in human buccal punch biopsies for use as pharmacodynamic biomarkers in drug development. *Br J Cancer* 2005; 93: 208–215.
3. Fleskens SJ, Takes RP, Otte-Höller I et al. Simultaneous assessment of DNA ploidy and biomarker expression in paraffin-embedded tissue sections. *Histopathology* 2010; 57: 14–26.
4. Sloan P, Bocking A. Oral cavity. In: Gray W, Kocjan G (eds) *Diagnostic Cytopathology*, 3rd edn. Edinburgh: Churchill Livingstone Elsevier, 2010: 253–264.
5. Remmerbach TW, Meyer-Ebrecht D, Aach T. et al. Toward a multimodal cell analysis of brush biopsies for the early detection of oral cancer. *Cancer* 2009; 117: 228–235.
6. Navone R, Burlo P, Pich A, Pentenero M, Broccoletti R, Marsico A, Gandolfo S. The impact of liquid-based oral cytology on the diagnosis of oral squamous dysplasia and carcinoma. *Cytopathology* 2007; 18: 356–360.
7. Klanrit P, Sperandio M, Brown AL, Shirlaw PJ, Challacombe SJ, Morgan PR, Odell EW. DNA ploidy in proliferative verrucous leukoplakia. *Oral Oncol* 2007; 43: 310–316.
8. Mehrotra R, Gupta A, Singh M, Ibrahim R. Application of cytology and molecular biology in diagnosing premalignant or malignant oral lesions. *Mol Cancer* 2006; 5: 11–86.
9. Kujan O, Oliver RJ, Khattab A, Roberts SA, Thakker N, Sloan P. Evaluation of a new binary system of grading oral epithelial dysplasia for prediction of malignant transformation. *Oral Oncol* 2006; 42: 987–993.
10. Abbey LM, Kaugars GE, Gunsolley JC et al. Intraexaminer and interexaminer reliability in the diagnosis of oral epithelial dysplasia. *Oral Surg Oral Med Oral Pathol* 1995; 80: 188–191.
11. Kujan O, Khattab A, Oliver RJ, Roberts SA, Thakker N, Sloan P. Why oral histopathology suffers inter-observer variability on grading oral epithelial dysplasia: an attempt to understand the sources of variation. *Oral Oncol* 2007; 43: 224–231.

12. Eversole LR. Dysplasia of the upper aerodigestive tract squamous epithelium *Head Neck Pathol* 2009; 3: 63–68.

13. Smith PA, Gray W. Cervical intraepithelial neoplasia and squamous cell carcinoma of the cervix. In: Gray W, Kocjan G (eds) *Diagnostic Cytopathology*, 3rd edn. Edinburgh: Churchill Livingstone Elsevier, 2010: 609–666.

14. McCredie MR, Sharples KJ, Paul C, Baranyai J, Medley G, Jones RW, Skegg DC. Natural history of cervical neoplasia and risk of invasive cancer in women with cervical intraepithelial neoplasia 3: a retrospective cohort study. *Lancet Oncol* 2008; 9: 425–434.

15. Barnes I, Eveson J, Reichart P, Sidransky D. *Pathology and Genetics of Head and Neck Tumours.IARC WHO Classification of Tumours*. Geneva: World Health Organisation, 2005.

16. Warnakulasuriya S, Reibel J, Bouquot J, Dabelsteen E. Oral epithelial dysplasia classification systems: predictive value, utility, weaknesses and scope for improvement. *J Oral Pathol Med* 2008; 37: 127–133.

17. Gale N, Michaels L, Luzar B, Poljak M, Zidar N, Fischinger J, Cardesa A. Current review on squamous intraepithelial lesions of the larynx. *Histopathology* 2009; 54: 639–656.

18. Kambic V, Lenart I. Our classification of hyperplasia of the laryngeal epithelium from the prognostic point of view. *J Fr Otorhinolaryngol Audiophonol Chir Maxillofac* 1971; 20: 1145–1150.

19. Gale N, Kambic V, Michaels L. et al. The Ljubljana classification: a practical strategy for the diagnosis of laryngeal precancerous lesions. *Adv Anat Pathol* 2000; 7: 240–251.

20. Izumo T. Oral premalignant lesions: from the pathological viewpoint. *Int J Clin Oncol* 2011; 16: 15–26.

21. Amarasinghe HK, Johnson NW, Lalloo R, Kumaraarachchi M, Warnakulasuriya S. Derivation and validation of a risk-factor model for detection of oral potentially malignant disorders in populations with high prevalence. *Br J Cancer* 2010; 103: 303–309.

22. Goodson ML, Robinson CM, Sloan P, Thomson PJ. Malignant transformation – how relevant is oral epithelial dysplasia? *Br J Oral Maxillofac Surg* 2010; 48 (Suppl 1): S19.

7 Management of Oral Precancer

Peter Thomson

Oral Precancer: Diagnosis and Management of Potentially Malignant Disorders, First Edition. Edited by Peter Thomson.
© 2012 John Wiley & Sons, Ltd. Published 2012 by John Wiley & Sons, Ltd.

Introduction

Having established both a clinical and then a histopathological diagnosis for an oral potentially malignant disorder in a patient, one of the principal difficulties in determining a management strategy is the lack of agreed and defined treatment protocols. Treatments are rarely evidence-based and are strongly influenced by individual clinician preferences and skill. There is a lack of clinically relevant randomised controlled trials, and most evidence is based upon cohort or observational studies.

Similarly, there are no universally agreed objectives of treatment interventions, although it is sensible to assume that there is a consensus view that prevention of oral cancer is a fundamental priority. The natural history of oral precancer remains ill defined and unpredictable, however, so that uncertainty inevitably haunts clinical management decisions. It is thus important for us to define pertinent management goals in attempting to treat oral precancer and a proposed summary of these are listed in Box 7.1. We have already seen that accurate diagnosis may not always be straightforward, but the ability to recognise the presence of early malignant change within lesions, together with the removal of dysplastic tissue and the prevention of further precancer disease, should be regarded as essential prerequisites for a successful management technique.

As detailed in Chapter 6, it is very important to ensure that we obtain as accurate and definitive a histopathological diagnosis for precancer patients as possible and it now seems clear that excision of precancer lesions in their entirety is necessary to establish this. Small, incisional biopsies for obvious reasons may not always be truly representative of the entire potentially malignant disorder [1,2].

Whilst formal surgical excision is carried out in order to remove all clinically apparent dysplastic tissue, it is extremely important to note that in nearly 10% of excised precancer lesions, microinvasive or frankly early invasive carcinomas are also identified unexpectedly on histological examination, presumably at a pathological stage when otherwise clinically undetectable [3]. It is thus obvious that, whilst the principal dilemma in oral precancer management strategies has always been whether to observe patients or to intervene and offer treatment, the recognition that a truly definitive diagnosis requires excision biopsy of the entire visible lesion places the emphasis in modern treatment protocols firmly upon surgical intervention.

In this chapter we will review the management techniques that have been proposed for oral precancer treatment (Box 7.2). We will also discuss in some

---

Box 7.1 Management goals in treating oral precancer.

- Accurate diagnosis
- Early recognition of malignancy
- Removal of dysplastic mucosa
- Prevention of recurrent or further disease
- Prevention of malignant transformation
- Minimal patient morbidity

Box 7.2   Treatment modalities for oral precancer.

- Risk factor identification and elimination
- Clinical observation
- Medical treatment
- Surgical excision

detail our preferred option of interventional laser surgery, which appears to be both an appropriate diagnostic tool and an efficacious treatment modality.

Risk factor modification

It is difficult to obtain meaningful figures for malignant transformation rates for precancers in the current literature, with quoted figures for the development of oral squamous cell carcinoma varying between 0.13% and 36.4% [3]. For leukoplakia, which is worldwide the commonest oral potentially malignant disorder, a figure of around 1% has been quoted as an overall annual transformation rate [1]. Widely disparate data such as these clearly have very limited use in discussing prognosis and behaviour with individual patients and certainly do not help in dealing with the myriad of potentially malignant lesions that present in the clinical situation.

Of more pragmatic benefit, therefore, is to try to identify which patients are at 'high risk' of malignant disease compared with those more likely to be 'low-risk' individuals. High-risk lesions, in other words those demonstrating severe dysplasia or carcinoma in situ, have been quoted to progress to cancer in up to 80% of cases. Low-risk lesions, showing at worst only mild dysplasia, tend to progress in less than 15% of cases.

As we have seen, however, such risk stratification is more difficult than might appear obvious at first sight. This is because a 'high-risk' patient is not just simply an older individual with a long history of smoking and alcohol use presenting, for example, with severely dysplastic leukoplakia in the floor of the mouth. An unpredictable 'high risk' may also affect young patients, particularly those with no demonstrable risk factor behaviour and can apply equally to mucosal lesions demonstrating sometimes quite minimal dysplasia.

There remains a surprising level of ignorance in the general population regarding mouth cancer and its causes. Any management protocol must therefore begin with education of patients about the aetiology of oral cancer and the importance of both recognising and then eliminating risk factors. In the vast majority of cases, of course, this relates primarily to tobacco and alcohol use, and it is disheartening how often patients fail to stop smoking or reduce their alcohol intake following diagnosis and treatment [4,5].

Smoking cessation

Tobacco smoking, primarily of cigarettes, is well documented as the principal aetiological agent in oral cancer development and there is a recognised dose–response relationship between increasing cancer risk and the amount and duration of tobacco use. Patients can usually estimate the number of cigarettes or amount of tobacco they smoke daily, although it is likely that they may underestimate this, either consciously or quite often subconsciously, when self-reporting to clinicians.

There is evidence that brief health care interventions can be effective in educating patients about the risks of tobacco smoking, and we have clearly shown that formal stopping smoking regimes can be very useful in precancer patients. However, these interventions are most effective when dedicated smoking cessation advisers attend clinics as members of the specialist dysplasia team [4]. Patients who try to stop smoking without formal cessation advice, who do not use nicotine replacement therapy to prevent acute withdrawal symptoms, or who have no regular contact with a dedicated cessation advisor are statistically highly unlikely to achieve long-term quitting.

It is salutary to note that nearly three-quarters of smoking patients treated for potentially malignant disorders remain as persistent smokers 5 years after their initial diagnoses. This not only risks further precancerous lesion development but also puts them at increased risk of malignant transformation [4].

In addition to tobacco smoking, as we have already seen, the use of smokeless tobacco is also an important risk factor but varies considerably worldwide, being particularly prominent in India and the southern states of the USA. In some parts of Sweden and Norway it is used as snus, which is a moist tobacco that is held under the upper lip and then sucked. In the UK smokeless tobacco is primarily seen as the classic betel quid in Asian communities and is composed of chewing tobacco mixed with areca nut, slaked lime and betel. People who use smokeless tobacco absorb similar amounts of nicotine and are as equally dependent as smokers. Advice on stopping the use of smokeless tobacco, behavioural therapy and the treatment of nicotine withdrawal symptoms are all thus equally important as treatment modalities in these patients as in their smoking counterparts [6].

Alcohol counselling

Assessing and then attempting to modify risk factor behaviour is integral to any management protocol for potentially malignant disorders. In relation to alcohol use it is complicated by patients' subjective and potentially unreliable estimates of self-reported intake and is also, of course, confounded by the concomitant use of tobacco [5]. Whilst it is undoubtedly true that most patients presenting with oral potentially malignant lesions are either current or ex-smokers, there is a small minority who have never smoked.

Controversy exists about whether alcohol alone increases precancerous transformation, but there is clear evidence that alcohol availability and consumption are both rising in most populations worldwide. It is probably within cohorts of patients who have never smoked that the role of alcohol is most significant. This effect of alcohol, however, is probably most likely to affect patients who consume alcohol both regularly and excessively. It is most likely that it is the overall amount that is drunk rather than the use of any individual type of alcohol that is most relevant.

Separating the complex interactions and observed synergistic effects between tobacco and alcohol use in oral precancer patients is probably impossible and the reality is such that the majority of patients usually consume both.

Attempts to establish more objective estimates of alcohol use may, however, be of value in precancer management. We investigated a cohort of 54 smokers presenting with new, single dysplastic oral lesions and demonstrated that an objective mean corpuscular red blood cell volume greater than 100 fl, as recorded in routine preoperative blood tests, corresponded with both a patient self-reporting of alcohol intake in excess of 28 units per week, and also an increased severity of dysplasia seen in their presenting oral lesions [5]. How successful individual patient counselling and advice to reduce alcohol intake is in influencing oral precancer outcomes is difficult to assess. However, it was disappointing to note that all 54 patients in our cohort study continued to drink alcohol following interventional laser treatment. Indeed, we also observed a significantly increased risk of further precancer disease developing in patients who continued with a high level of alcohol intake post-surgery [5].

Nonetheless, identification of patients with excessive alcohol intake offers important opportunities for education and health care interventions and should be encouraged in all potentially malignant disorder cases.

Modification of other risk factors

In non-smoking patients and those with low alcohol consumption, the importance and relevance of other risk factors may require further elucidation. The type of risk factors requiring attention here include deficiencies in dietary intake of fresh fruit and vegetables, a possible influence for human papillomavirus (HPV) and oral sexual behaviour, together with a number of background medical conditions, such as immunosuppression, all of which may influence both dysplasia development and disease progression.

It may not always be possible to reduce the significance or alter the course of these rather disparate disease influences, but it is certainly important to be able to identify them and recognise their relevance to individual patient care pathways.

Observation versus intervention

Traditionally, clinical observation protocols – which essentially comprised initial lesion recognition and diagnosis, photography, routine oral inspection and patient monitoring – have been the mainstay of oral potentially malignant disorder management. Unfortunately this has led in many cases to, effectively, a passive observation of cancer development in a previously identified precancer patient. This seems both self-defeating and highly inadequate as a 21st century patient care pathway. Thus, it is hardly surprising that interventional management protocols have developed to try to prevent such disastrous transformations and most authors now recommend active treatment, rather than clinical observation, for all oral precancer lesions [1].

A period of clinical observation may, however, be appropriate for patients with low-grade dysplasia who stop smoking, who are prepared to address other relevant risk factor behaviours, and who are willing and able to attend for regular clinical review. It is recognised that in many cases lesions may improve and regress following smoking cessation, but it is important that this is carefully monitored.

Failure of precancer lesions to resolve may mean that the patient has actually been unable to stop smoking or, perhaps of more significance, the recognition of persistent disease in the absence of smoking may indicate irreversible dysplastic change. As a result this may well be an important patient subgroup in which to reconsider surgical intervention.

In the absence of appropriate randomised controlled clinical trials we retrospectively reviewed two of our patient cohorts over a 3-year period. One cohort was a laser excision group of 78 patients exhibiting high-grade single dysplastic lesions and the other an observed group of 39 patients with low-grade dysplasia. During the follow-up period 64% of laser patients showed complete clinical resolution of their disease whilst, perhaps unsurprisingly, only 23% of observed only lesions resolved [7].

Whilst the above is a useful comparative, observational 'snap shot', there is a clear need for proper randomised controlled trials with long-term patient follow up to investigate such treatment decisions and resultant clinical outcomes in more detail.

Medical treatment

A variety of medical interventions have been attempted through the years to treat precancer lesions, utilising both local and systemic chemopreventive agents. These have included the use of carotenoids, vitamins A, C and E, bleomycin and more recently cyclo-oxygenase inhibitors. The types of drugs that have been utilised, their proposed mechanisms of action and any recognised side effects consequent upon their use are summarised in Table 7.1.

Systematic reviews of medical interventions for oral precancer have, unfortunately, proved unhelpful in determining realistic management strategies and

Agent	Mode of action	Side effects
Carotenoids		
Beta carotene (vitamin A precursor)	Antioxidant	Yellow skin discolouration, headaches, muscle pain
Lycopene	Antioxidant	None
Vitamins		
Ascorbic acid (vitamin C)	Antioxidant	None
Alpha tocoferol (vitamin E)	Antioxidant	None
Retinoic acid (vitamin A): 13-cis-retinoic acid	Keratin production; epithelial cell growth and differentiation; collagen matrix production	Dermatitis, teratogenic, headaches, muscle pain, xerostomia, dizziness
Isotretinoin Tretinoin		
Fenretinide (vitamin A analogue)	Apoptosis induction	None
Bleomycin	Cytotoxic antibiotic	Stomatitis, alopecia, skin pruritus and vesiculation
Ketorolac	NSAID	Gastroduodenal irritation
Celecoxib	Selective COX-2 inhibitor	Cardiovascular thrombosis
Tea/green tea	Anti-angiogenesis	Insomnia, nervousness

NSAID, non-steroidal anti-inflammatory drug.

Table 7.1 Medical treatments in oral precancer management.

very few relevant randomised controlled trials exist in the literature [8]. It is also disheartening to note that very little benefit has ever been shown from such medical treatments. There is no evidence, for example, of any effective long-term clinical resolution, no significant prevention of malignant transformation of lesions and no reduction in either disease incidence or recurrence compared with observation alone or placebo treatment [8–10].

Furthermore, many of the clinical trials undertaken were carried out on small numbers of patients over short study durations, usually with cases followed up for only a few months rather than years post treatment, which is necessary to identify relevant malignant transformation risks. Where clinical improvement was noted during the trial, lesions often worsened again on cessation of therapy and, because no clear definitions of treatment goals or end points were established, the overall significance of many of these treatments remains unclear. Of similar concern was the observation that numerous side effects of medical treatments were common (Table 7.1). These, to a greater or lesser extent, affected the majority of study participants, sometimes interfering with compliance and prompting subjects to withdraw from treatments.

Finally, and perhaps of most significance, is the fact that all pre-treatment diagnoses relied entirely upon incisional biopsy histopathological classification, which we now recognise, of course, as only a provisional diagnosis. As whole lesion examination is deemed necessary for definitive histopathological diagnosis, it is not unreasonable to view medical treatments as fundamentally flawed therapies applied to diseased mucosa in the absence of definitive pathological diagnoses [1,2].

Photodynamic therapy (PDT) is a particularly specialised and emerging form of medical intervention, which relies on cellular destruction by a cold photochemical reaction following activation of a photosensitising drug, such as aminolevulinic acid or temoporfin, by low-power visible light. This technique has been advocated by some as a non-invasive oral precancer treatment although it remains primarily a tool for palliative treatment of advanced squamous cell carcinoma of the head and neck. A number of observational studies have reported variable success rates using PDT to treat oral leukoplakia. However, there has been inconsistent reporting regarding recurrent disease and to date only limited, between 3 and 6 months, or no follow-up data [10].

There thus remains a fundamental lack of randomised controlled trials for non-surgical treatment of oral potentially malignant disorders. Those that do exist in the literature show no satisfactory evidence of effective treatment of individual precancer lesions or prevention of oral malignancy.

One feature that is agreed by most authors, and which is really central to oral precancer management, is that regular patient follow up and repeated detailed clinical examination remains mandatory for all potentially malignant disorder patients irrespective of the mode of proposed treatment [10].

Surgical treatment

Surgical treatment of oral potentially malignant disorders is clearly designed to prevent malignant transformation by removing lesions and thus freeing patients from the risk of cancer at affected sites. Critics of surgical intervention observe that not only is there little evidence to support the above hypothesis, but that no randomised controlled trials of surgical intervention, particularly one that includes a no treatment or placebo arm, have ever been carried out [8].

Nonetheless, surgery remains the first choice in oral precancer management by most specialists, especially for lesions exhibiting high-grade dysplasia [11,12].

Initial surgical interventions relied upon scalpel excision and primary closure of defects and mucosal or split skin grafting for larger defects. Neither proved popular with patients or clinicians, primarily due to localised postoperative contracture and deformity and the frequent failure of skin grafts to take in the oral environment. Management of widespread, multifocal disease with such techniques was virtually impossible.

Cryotherapy is a specialised technique involving the localised destruction of diseased tissue by the surgical application of extreme cold usually via liquid nitrogen. This has been popular in the past for treating oral lesions but is less commonly used today and is actually a highly unsatisfactory technique which is not recommended for precancer or cancer treatment. Not only does significant postoperative pain and swelling result from the tissue damage consequent upon cryotherapy, but also potentially malignant lesions are rarely successfully or completely destroyed and, of course, no excision biopsy is undertaken to establish a definitive diagnosis. This potentially leaves partially treated dysplastic tissue in situ, which may then be 'stimulated', presumably by extensive tissue damage, to more aggressive clinical behaviour. Interestingly, both high recurrence and increased malignant transformation rates have been reported following the use of cryotherapy for precancer, which supports these concerns [9].

Interventional laser surgery

Interventional laser therapies have evolved following demonstrable failure of observational or medical therapies and the limitations of conventional surgery in treating oral precancer disease. A number of cohort studies have demonstrated an important role for laser surgery as both a diagnostic tool and a treatment modality in the management of potentially malignant disorders [2,13,14].

The term laser is an acronym for 'light amplification by stimulated emission of radiation'. The laser device essentially emits a monochromatic, coherent wave of light energy that is then delivered to the target tissue via fibreoptic systems, hollow waveguides or a series of articulated arms and mirrors. Figure 7.1 illustrates the laser device and articulated arm system of a standard carbon dioxide (CO_2) surgical laser, as seen prepared for use in the operating

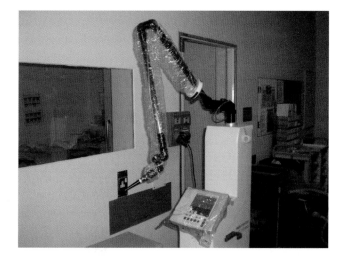

Figure 7.1 Carbon dioxide laser prepared for use in the operating theatre, demonstrating the articulated arm arrangement linked by freely moveable joints and containing precisely aligned mirrors that maintain the laser beam in a central position until it reaches the handpiece.

theatre. This type of laser uses sealed CO_2 gas as the active medium to generate laser light in the mid-infrared range at 10 600 nm. As this is near the spectroscopic absorption peak for water, all oral soft tissues successfully interact with the CO_2 laser beam.

A photothermal reaction occurs when laser light interacts with the target tissue. Between 60 and 100°C, this produces coagulation which facilitates either localised haemostasis or tissue necrosis. At and above 100°C, when water boils, there is vapourisation which allows the surgeon to incise tissue, and to either resect or ablate lesions.

Safety regulations govern the use of surgical lasers and include wearing wavelength-specific protective eyewear, using a high-volume smoke evacuation system and restricting access to the laser surgery area.

Introduction of the CO_2 laser to oral surgery practice in the 1970s revolutionised interventional therapy allowing convenient, effective and reproducible treatments. Box 7.3 lists a number of specific advantages of laser surgery. With preserved function of oral tissues and the ability to re-apply laser therapy to previously treated areas, CO_2 laser surgery is now the preferred treatment in many medical institutes.

In recent years a variety of different types of laser have been introduced into surgical practice, such as the neodymium;yttrium–aluminium–garnet (Nd : YAG) laser, or in combination with potassium–titanyl–phosphate as the KTP laser, or argon and diode lasers. They all have their individual advocates, although there is no evidence to suggest that any one of these is more effective than another.

While the CO_2 laser has certainly been utilised and studied the most in clinical practice, it is probably the experience and skill of the individual surgeon in identifying the site and extent of oral lesions and in determining excision margins appropriately at the time of surgery that is of most relevance to clinical outcome.

Surgical techniques

We have used the CO_2 laser extensively in the treatment of potentially malignant disorders and recommend it as the optimal oral precancer treatment.

Box 7.3 Advantages of interventional laser surgery

- Rapid, precise tissue dissection and lesion excision
- Minimal damage to adjacent normal tissue
- Haemostasis
- Postoperative analgesia
- Definitive histopathological diagnosis
- Low morbidity and minimal swelling with low infection rates
- Rapid healing
- Reduced oral mucosal scarring and contracture
- Excellent patient acceptance
- Facilitates multiple or repeated treatment

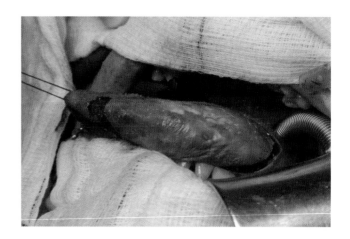

Figure 7.2 Saline-soaked swabs are placed around the facial soft tissues to prevent inadvertent laser damage during surgery. In this case a lateral tongue lesion is being excised. Note the armoured endotracheal tube, which is just visible posteriorly in the oral cavity behind the tongue.

It is useful, therefore, to describe in some detail the technique of such interventional surgery. Laser treatment may be carried out using local anaesthesia, primarily for medically compromised patients or the removal of small, circumscribed lesions in the anterior oral cavity. It can also be performed under endotracheal general anaesthesia, which facilitates the excision of large and/or posteriorly sited precancer lesions.

In the latter case, to avoid the devastasting complication of airway fire, specialised laser-safe endotracheal tubes are utilised. These are airtight and covered by a reflective metal exterior. Damp throat packs and similarly moistened swabs are also used as additional layers of airway and facial soft tissue protection. Figure 7.2 illustrates both the armoured endotracheal tube in place and the damp swabs surrounding the face in a patient undergoing a general anaesthetic laser excision of a dysplastic lateral tongue leukoplakia.

Box 7.4 summarises a number of important considerations when interventional laser surgery is undertaken utilising general anaesthesia techniques.

Box 7.4 Features of anaesthetic management and intra-oral laser surgery.*

Preoperative assessment
- General systemic enquiry and airway assessment

Monitoring
- ECG, non-invasive blood pressure, SaO_2, end tidal CO_2, end tidal inhalational agent concentration, minimum alveolar concentration

Induction
- Fentanyl, propofol, atracurium, oxygen, air, servoflurane, antibiotics, dexamethasone, IV fluids

Intubation
- Mallinckrodt laser-flex orotracheal tube (flexible stainless steel hose with plastic segment at the distal end and two cuffs); the distal cuff is inflated first with normal saline to stop audible leak, followed by the proximal cuff
- Before inflating the cuff, the tube is positioned in the mouth on the opposite side to the lesion to be operated upon

Protection
- Laryngopharynx and oropharynx are packed around the tube with normal saline-soaked gauze pack
- Remaining length of pack is wrapped around portion of tube in the mouth and outside
- Surgeon covers exposed face, endotracheal tube, anaesethetic tubing and connections with wet swabs
- Patient's eyes are closed with tape and covered with saline-soaked eye pads

Maintenance
- Intermittent positive pressure ventilation with air, oxygen and servoflurane
- Maintain SaO_2 above 95% and end tidal CO_2 at 5–6 kPa

Intraoperative analgesia
- Local anaesthetic infiltration at lesion site by surgeon
- IV paracetamol, ketorolac and/or morphine

Extubation
- Inhalation agent discontinued
- Throat pack removed, oropharyngeal suction and reversal of neuromuscular blockade
- 100% oxygen adminstered
- Once spontaneous breathing is established, cuffs are deflated of saline and patient is extubated in a 20–30° head-up position

Possible complications
- Airway damage due to inhalation of laser plumes or smoke
- Airway fire
- Burns
- Extubation stridor
- Sore throat

CO_2, carbon dioxide; ECG, electrocardiogram; IV, intravenous.
Courtesy of Dr Remani Wariyar, Department of Anaesthesia, Royal Victoria Infirmary, Newcastle upon Tyne Hospitals NHS Foundation Trust.

Buccal mucosa surgery Whilst the general principles of laser surgery are the same throughout the oral cavity, there are slight differences in technique dependent upon the anatomical site. The following description outlines the excision of a buccal mucosal erythroleukoplakia that exhibited severe dysplasia on incisional biopsy. This lesion is illustrated in Figure 7.3.

The CO_2 laser is used for this surgery, with procedures performed using power levels between 10 and 15 W. Surgical excision is carried out using a hand-held delivery device (Figure 7.4) with a laser spot size of 1 mm diameter. The handpiece is provided with a helium–neon-aiming beam, facilitating guidance to the target. An evacuation system is necessary to remove both smoke and debris from the surgical site.

The single pulse mode is used to outline the resection margins, which are ideally situated at least 5 mm outside the apparent clinical margins of the target lesion.

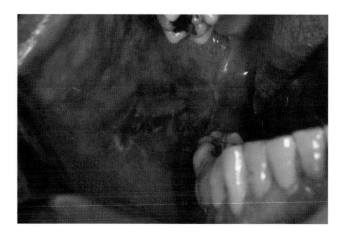

Figure 7.3 Erythroleukoplakic buccal lesion that showed severe dysplasia histopathologically on incision biopsy examination. (Figures 7.3–7.8 shown the same patient.)

These markings are shown in Figure 7.5, although it is recognised that the placement of excision margins in this way is based upon the rather subjective judgement of the operating surgeon. In order to improve objectivity and to try to ensure complete lesion excision with dysplasia-free margins, VELscope® imaging, as described in Chapter 5, may be used as an adjunct during surgery to confirm or delineate further the extent of abnormal mucosa. The use of the VELscope in the operating theatre immediately before laser surgery is shown in Figure 7.6.

The pulse marks are then connected using the laser in a continuous mode, deepening the incision to approximately 5 mm in the submucosal plane. This is

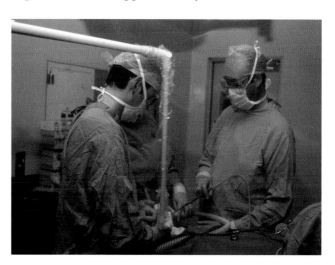

Figure 7.4 Use of the CO_2 laser in the operating theatre. The handpiece is directed to the intra-oral operative field by the surgeon.

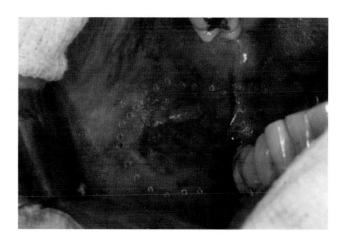

Figure 7.5 Marking out excision margins, which are usually placed at least 5 mm outside the visible extent of the mucosal lesion, using a 'single shot', slightly defocused laser beam.

(A)

(B)

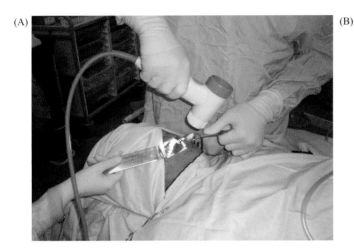

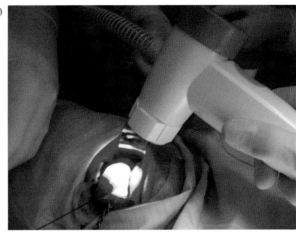

Figure 7.6 Tissue autofluorescence, here showing the VELscope in use in the theatre (A), may aid in visualising the full extent of dysplastic mucosal lesions (B) thus helping to determine definitive excision margins immediately prior to laser surgery.

illustrated in Figure 7.7, which demonstrates the extent of the mucosal lesion which is to be removed. The depth of excision is affected not only by the anatomical site – such that it is usually less when involving thin floor of mouth tissue or when mucosa is resected overlying alveolar bone – but it is also significantly influenced by the extent of dysplasia. More severe dysplasias, for example, are more likely to contain microinvasive or early invasive squamous cell carcinoma foci. It is therefore advisable to carry out the resection at a deeper level.

The whole specimen is then resected by undercutting at a constant depth (Figure 7.8). This photograph demonstrates both the submucosal tissue dissection and the underlying buccinator muscle, which lies immediately beneath the excision specimen at this site.

Following excision, the surgical bed and all the peripheral margins are vapourised using a defocused laser beam to eliminate residual disease and facilitate haemostasis. This defocusing is readily achieved by holding the laser handpiece further away from the surgical site. The appearance of the wound following this process is shown in Figure 7.9. It is well worth spending a few minutes on treating the wound base and all margins carefully and methodically at this point. This improves postoperative comfort, expedites healing and extends the treatment field several millimetres beyond the surgical excision zone.

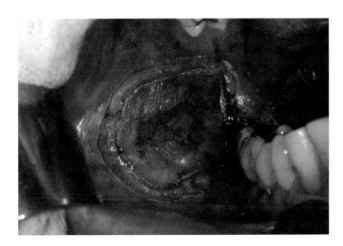

Figure 7.7 The pulse marks are connected using the laser in 'continuous' mode, which facilitates incision of the buccal tissue. The incision for this severe dysplasia resection is deepened to about 5 mm.

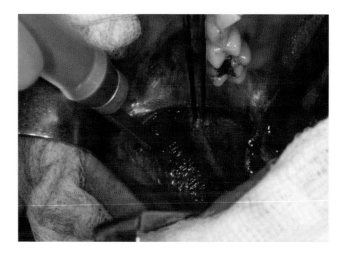

Figure 7.8 The dysplastic buccal mucosa is resected by undercutting at a constant depth, here showing a submucosal dissection and displaying the underlying buccinator muscle.

The excision specimen should be sutured at one or two points to aid later tissue orientation (Figure 7.10). It is then placed in formal saline solution prior to forwarding on to the pathology laboratory for histopathological analysis and establishment of a definitive diagnosis as discussed in Chapter 6.

There is little in the way of immediate postoperative pain, swelling or discomfort and patients are allowed to take clear fluids straight away if required, followed at least 2 hours later by a gradually increasing soft diet. Excised areas heal well by secondary intention, with a fibrinous cream-coloured coagulum forming over the wound within the first few days. This is followed by

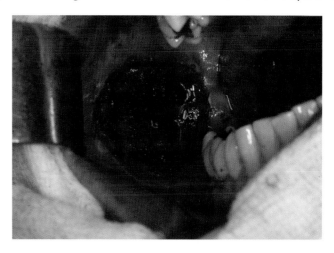

Figure 7.9 Following lesion excision, the surgical bed and all peripheral margins are vapourised using a defocused 'continuous' laser beam to eliminate residual mucosal disease at the margins and to facilitate haemostasis.

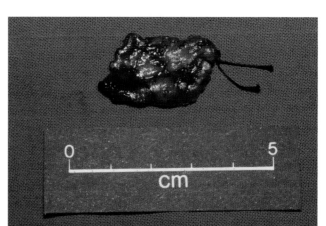

Figure 7.10 Mucosal excision specimen, showing a marking suture at the anterior resection margin to aid tissue orientation in the pathology laboratory.

re-epithelialisation from the surrounding wound edges, which is usually complete within 4–6 weeks.

Due to the effects of laser vapourisation, a lack of mechanical trauma during surgery and the absence of wound suturing, scarring is usually minimal and excellent aesthetic and functional results ensue. Figure 7.11 shows the appearance of healed buccal mucosa approximately 4 months post-laser excision of a dysplastic precancer lesion.

Figure 7.12 summarises a similar procedure for laser excision of a dysplastic leukoplakia arising more anteriorly from the labial commissure. In this case the anterior excision margin extends close to the vermilion border (Figure 7.12E).

Lateral tongue surgery Partial glossectomy by laser offers an excellent therapeutic tool for lateral tongue lesions. Figure 7.13 demonstrates laser excision of lateral tongue tissue for a severely dysplastic lesion. The surgical technique is carried out in a similar manner to the buccal and labial surgery outlined above.

Following excision, the wound is vapourised (Figure 7.14) to eliminate residual dysplastic disease and facilitate haemostasis and postoperative analgesia. Care should be taken, however, during the vapourisation phase as the lingual nerve often lies quite superficial along the side of the tongue and may be traumatised.

Figure 7.15 shows the tongue appearance 2 weeks after laser surgery demonstrating not only the creamy fibrinous coagulum but also the underlying pink and healthy granulation tissue that covers the wound base as part of the secondary intention healing process. By 3 months post laser, healing is normally complete and, as illustrated in Figure 7.16, there should be minimal scarring with good function. A further example of excellent post-laser healing of the posterolateral tongue is seen in Figure 7.17. It is thus clear that, following laser excision carried out in this way, there is no need for primary closure, skin grafting or flap reconstruction.

Due to the muscular nature of the tongue, the depth of lateral tongue resection can be varied much more than, for example, buccal mucosa or floor of mouth sites. This can be particularly useful when lesions exhibiting more severe dysplasia are treated and require more extensive tissue removal (Figure 7.18), although deeper excisions may cause more bleeding from divided tongue musculature. Careful and thorough use of diathermy is often required to ensure haemostasis before laser vapourisation is carried out.

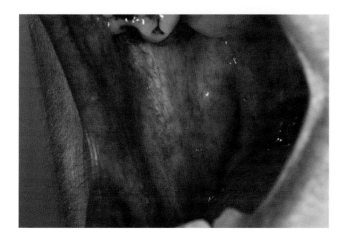

Figure 7.11 Buccal mucosal healing approximately 4 months following laser excision of a large dysplastic lesion, demonstrating minimal scarring and no restriction in mouth opening. (Not the same patient as shown in Figures 7.3–7.8.)

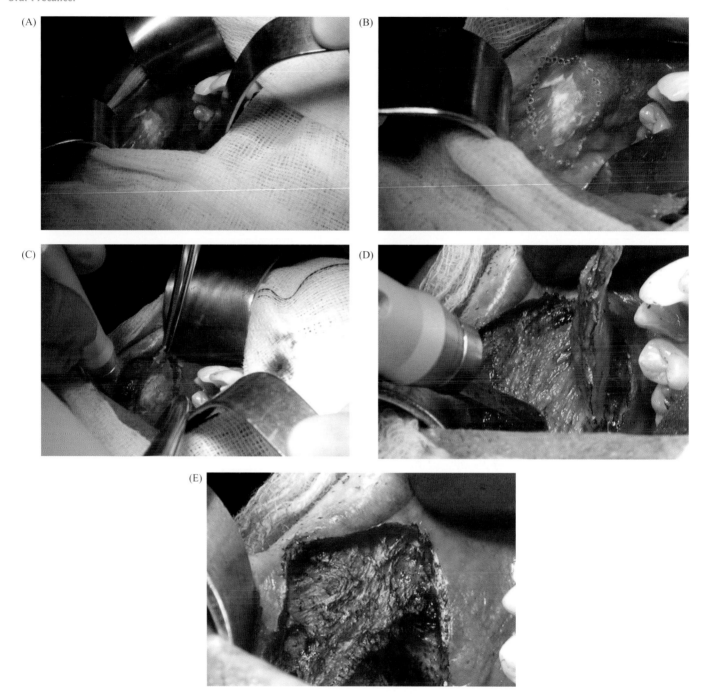

Figure 7.12 Illustration of a dysplastic leukoplakia arising at the labial commissure immediately prior to laser excision (A), the outline of the proposed resection margins (B), commencement of laser excision of the lesion (C), resection demonstrating the underlying buccinator muscle in the submucosal dissection plane (D), and post-laser excision vapourisation of all the wound margins (E).

Tongue dorsum surgery   The tongue dorsum is an unusual site for oral precancer lesions, but responds well to laser intervention. The gustatory mucosa (Figure 7.19), however, is relatively thick and requires both a deeper incision and the placement of a deeper undercutting layer to successfully raise the excision specimen. Healing is very rapid though with little in the way of scarring or functional impairment.

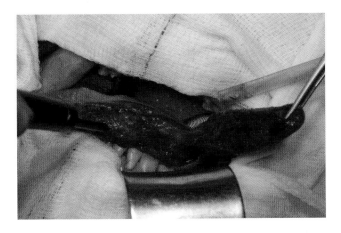

Figure 7.13 Partial glossectomy by laser, here excising a severely dysplastic mucosal lesion on the lateral border of the tongue (same patient as shown in Figure 7.2).

Ventral tongue surgery The mucosa on the ventral tongue surface, in contrast to the dorsum, is very thin. Figure 7.20 summarises laser excision of a dysplastic lesion arising on the ventral tongue mucosa. Beneath the thin mucosa lie the sublingual veins and the lingual nerve, all of which may be unavoidably damaged due to their proximity to the surface. To avoid troublesome bleeding both during and after surgery, it is often best to divide and ligate the veins at the

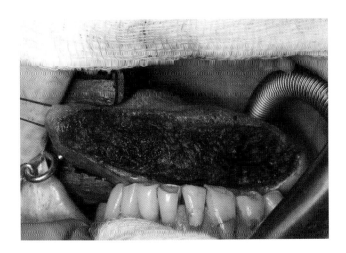

Figure 7.14 Following excision, the surgical bed and peripheral margins have been vapourised by defocused laser beam application.

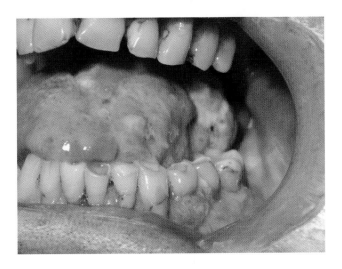

Figure 7.15 By 14 days, post-laser healing by secondary intention is well underway and a creamy fibrinous coating is evident together with underlying pink and healthy granulation tissue.

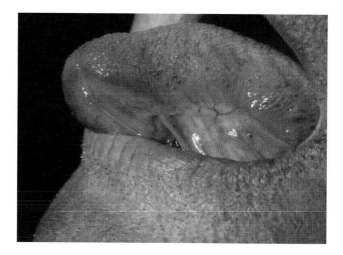

Figure 7.16 At 3 months, the tongue has healed well with minimal scarring, good appearance and excellent functional mobility.

commencement of the resection. Patients should be warned of the risk of lingual nerve dysaesthesia post surgery. Healing, however, is usually excellent with little in the way of scarring and contracture, and tongue mobility and speech are rarely significantly affected.

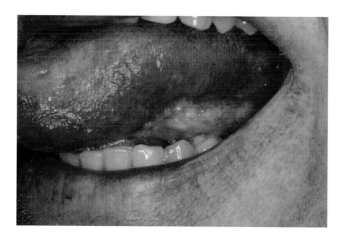

Figure 7.17 In this further example of lateral tongue surgery, typically good healing with minimal scarring is seen 6 months after laser excision of a more posteriorly sited leukoplakia.

(A) (B)

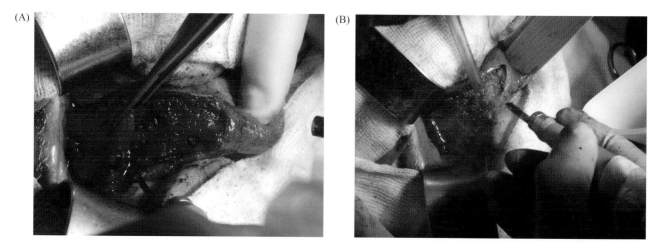

Figure 7.18 Laser excision of a severely dysplastic erythroplakia from the lateral tongue, undertaken at a deeper level and exposing more of the underlying tongue musculature (A), followed by defocused laser vapourisation to the wound margins (B).

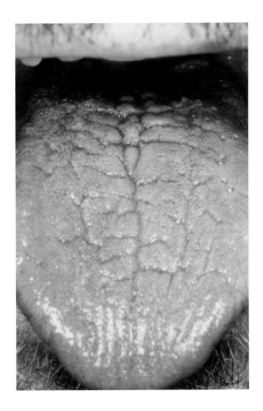

Figure 7.19 The gustatory mucosa on the tongue dorsum is thick and requires a deeper initial laser incision followed by undercutting at a deep layer to successfully raise the excision specimen.

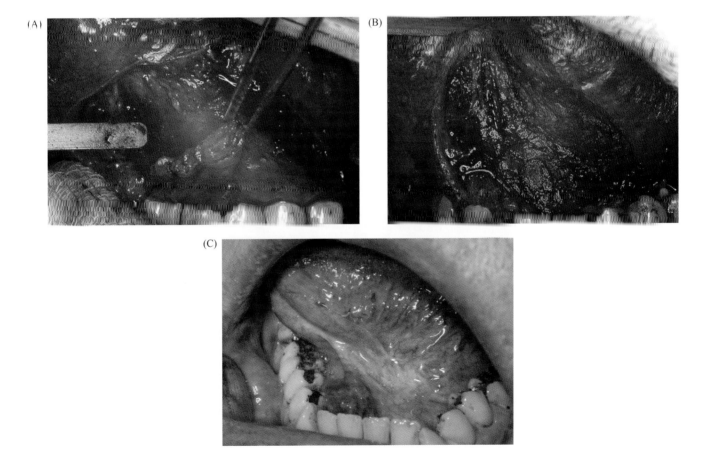

Figure 7.20 Laser excision of a moderately dysplastic leukoplakic lesion on the ventral tongue showing resection in progress (A), immediate post-excision vapourisation (B), and minimal scarring and good tongue mobility 3 months post treatment (C).

Floor of mouth surgery Surgical access to the floor of the mouth can sometimes be quite difficult in the dentate patient, particularly if the lower incisor teeth are retroclined. Similar to ventral tongue surgery, the procedure is complicated by important anatomical structures lying in the immediate submucosal tissues such as the submandibular ducts and sublingual veins anteriorly, and the sublingual salivary gland and lingual nerve which are sited more posteriorly.

Figure 7.21A shows the surgical technique for a floor of mouth resection, illustrated for clarity in an edentulous patient, whilst a prominent sublingual vein is demonstrated just before it is ligated and divided in Figure 7.21B. The immediate post-excision vapourisation appearance is seen in Figure 7.21C and the longer term postoperative healing is shown in Figure 7.21D.

Figure 7.22 illustrates anterior floor of mouth healing in a dentate patient 6 months after laser excision of a widespread, severely dysplastic lesion. There is more scarring evident in this example due to the requirement to excise both a large and deeper specimen. Nonetheless there remains excellent tongue mobility and good function with minimal morbidity. In Figure 7.23 good healing is demonstrated in the posterior floor of mouth region at around 6 months post-laser excision of a leukoplakic lesion. If excessive scarring occurs at this site it can lead to both tongue tethering and lingual nerve dysaesthesia.

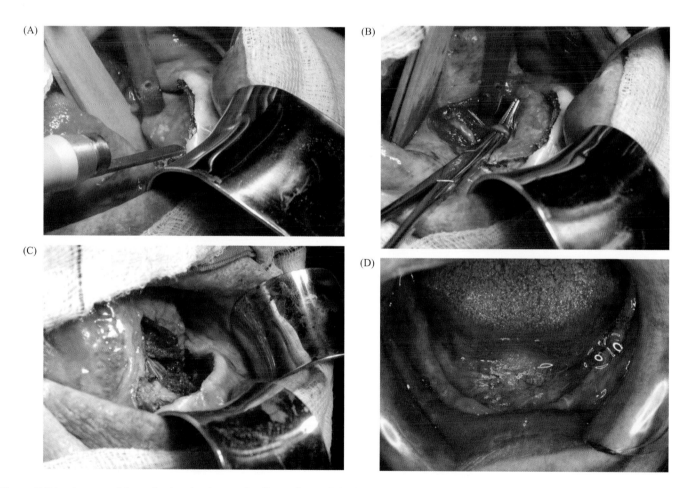

(A)   (B)   (C)   (D)

Figure 7.21   Laser excision of a dysplastic anterior floor of mouth lesion in an edentulous patient showing surgical resection in progress (A), dissection and then tying off of a prominent sublingual vein (B), post-excision vapourisation (C), and resultant excellent healing 3 months post laser with little scarring and no tongue tethering (D).

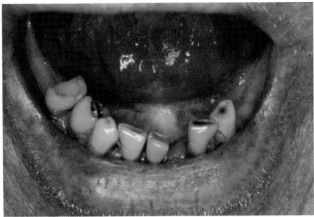

Figure 7.22 Anterior floor of mouth healing in a dentate patient 6 months after laser excision of a widespread, severely dysplastic erythroleukoplakia. Although there is evidence of more scarring here, due to the requirement for a larger excision specimen, good tongue mobility is preserved.

Soft palate and faucial pillar surgery   Despite their posterior location, surgery at these sites is usually straightforward although good mouth opening is required for optimal access. Careful positioning of both the endotracheal tube and the throat pack are important considerations in the anaesthetised patient. Figure 7.24A illustrates a non-homogeneous leukoplakia arising on the soft palate mucosa, whilst Figure 7.24B shows the immediate post-laser excision and vapourisation appearance. In Figure 7.25 laser excision of a dysplastic erythroleukoplakic lesion on the soft palate has been extended to include

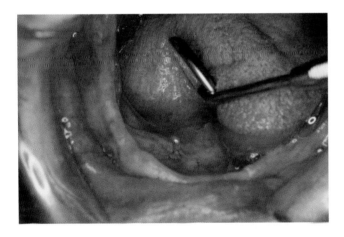

Figure 7.23 Post-laser healing 6 months after the excision of a more posteriorly sited floor of mouth leukoplakia in an edentulous patient.

(A)   (B)

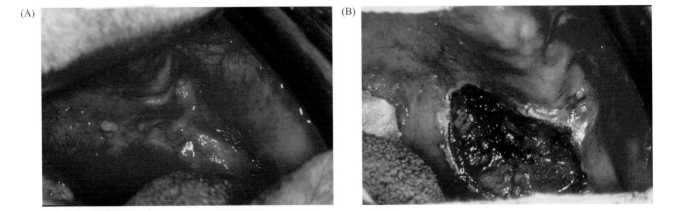

Figure 7.24 Diffuse, non-homogeneous leukoplakia arising on the soft palate mucosa (A) and the appearance following laser excision and vapourisation (B).

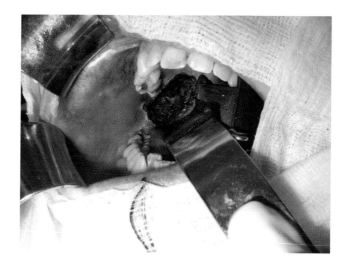

Figure 7.25 The soft palate excision has been extended along the pterygomandibular raphe towards the retromolar region. This is the appearance immediately following post-laser excision vapourisation.

abnormal mucosa along the anterior pillar of the fauces and pterygomandibular raphe, extending inferiorly towards the retromolar trigone.

As in most oral sites, careful retraction to place the tissues under tension is important to facilitate ease of mucosal resection. This is shown quite well in Figure 7.26, where the buccal tissues are being held under tension by a retractor to facilitate both access to the pterygomandibular raphe area, and also to allow extension of the resection out further towards the buccal mucosa.

The principal difficulty of carrying out laser excision surgery in the posterior oral cavity and oropharynx is to avoid creating soft palate defects or extensive haemorrhage in the palatoglossal folds and tonsillar regions which can sometimes be quite difficult to control. For the treatment of less severe dysplasia, therefore, it may be acceptable to ablate posterior lesions at these sites rather than formally excising them. However, this specific laser surgery technique has a number of disadvantages and will be discussed in more detail later.

Hard palate, gingiva and alveolar mucosa surgery At all of these sites, where the mucosa is tightly bound down to the underlying periosteum, it can be difficult to establish acceptable planes of laser dissection without creating large areas of denuded bone which inevitable heal extremely slowly. As with soft palate lesions, it may be best to consider superficial lesion ablation rather than excision. Overall, however, laser surgery offers the significant advantage of formally excising and thus removing the entire visible precancer lesion. This then facilitates subsequent definitive histopathological analysis and diagnosis.

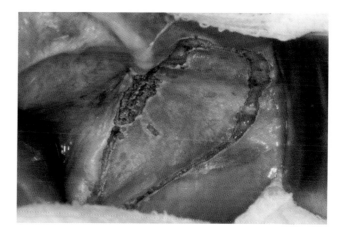

Figure 7.26 The buccal tissues are being held under tension to facilitate both access to the faucial pillars and to allow extension of the laser resection out towards the buccal mucosa.

Complete lesion excision does appear to help reduce malignant transformation at the site of the original lesion presentation. In addition, in approximately 10% of our patients, it has also identified unexpected early invasive squamous cell carcinoma histopathologically at an otherwise clinically undetectable stage [3].

A more detailed analysis of clinical outcome following treatment of potentially malignant lesions will be discussed in Chapter 8, whilst the important subject of malignant transformation and carcinoma development is reviewed in Chapter 9.

Laser excision versus ablation

It is important to clearly distinguish between two different laser surgery techniques: *laser excision* and *laser ablation*. In excision, the laser is used essentially as a 'scalpel', as described and illustrated above, to formally remove entire lesions from the oral mucosa. This is in contradistinction to ablation where the surface mucosa only is destroyed – to a varying depth selected by the surgeon and dependent upon the pathological lesion being treated – using a defocused laser beam. An example of laser ablation is shown in Figure 7.27, which illustrates the destruction of a small patch of mildly dysplastic floor of mouth mucosa.

Laser ablation is not routinely recommended because tissue is not excised for histopathological examination and the most abnormal basal epithelium may be left in situ. There may even be a theoretical risk of such intervention worsening the disease progress, particularly in the most severe dysplasias, stirring up further proliferative activity during epithelial regeneration in already dysplastic tissue, which may thus encourage malignant transformation.

Ablative techniques do have a small role, however, particularly in treating non-dysplastic or mildly dysplastic lesions on tightly bound-down alveolar or gingival tissue where excision may lead to areas of slow or non-healing mucosa, producing painful areas of denuded and ultimately non-vital alveolar bone.

And, as discussed above, there may also be a small role for laser ablation at certain oral sites such as the soft palate or labial mucosa, where tissue excision may lead to significant functional or cosmetic disturbance.

(A)

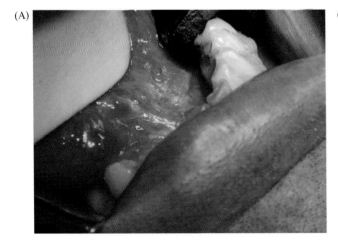

(B)

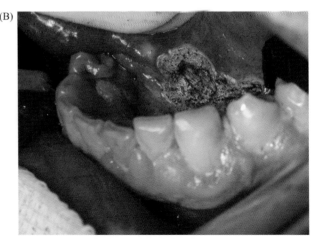

Figure 7.27   In this patient, a small patch of mildly dysplastic leukoplakia arising on the floor of mouth (A) was treated by laser ablation rather than formal laser excision (B).

Management of multiple lesion disease with laser surgery

The presence of multiple or widespread oral disease poses a significant management problem for precancer patients. This is because it is rarely possible to treat or excise all the abnormal mucosa and there are known to be both unpredictable and high rates of malignant transformation [15]. Figure 7.28 illustrates the extensive mucosal involvement seen in a patient with multifocal oral leukoplakia.

Due to inherently unstable oral mucosa in these cases, the ability to identify the most severe areas of dysplasia via field mapping techniques is useful to help direct laser surgery to the most significantly diseased tissue. In a series of 16 consecutive, new patients with multiple lesion disease, we reported on incisional biopsies carried out at 70 oral sites. These biopsies helped identify and then facilitate laser excision of the 11 lesions harbouring the most severe dysplasia. Lesions exhibiting more significant dysplasia were seen to affect particularly the faucial pillars, floor of mouth and ventral tongue sites [16].

Rationalisation of therapeutic intervention to the most significantly affected intra-oral sites in this way is a major step forward in the management of multiple lesion disease. However it remains unclear whether there are any differences in outcome between lesions that present either synchronously or metachronously, and whether the total area involved in mucosal abnormality influences the long-term treatment response [16].

Nonetheless, field mapping can certainly be recommended for multiple lesion patients. It is also possible that the use of diagnostic adjuncts such as fluorescence imaging and brush biopsies for exfoliative cytology may aid in the clinical assessment and longer term management of this difficult subgroup of precancer patients.

Complications of laser surgery

The use of interventional laser surgery has helped to rationalise treatment decisions in oral precancer management and is a safe, reliable and predictable therapy. Like all surgical interventions, however, there are possible complications of its use and it is important for us to consider these in assessing the overall efficacy of laser treatment.

(A)   (B)

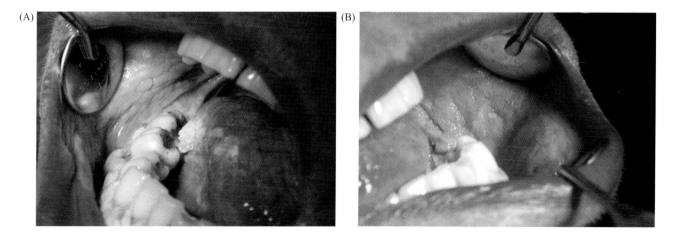

Figure 7.28 (A, B) This patient has widespread multifocal dysplastic leukoplakia, showing extensive involvement of the buccal mucosa, mandibular buccal gingiva and both lateral and dorsal tongue sites.

Complications are generally defined as unwanted events that may render surgery more difficult, intricate or involved than expected. Complications may arise in the immediate preoperative phase usually because of underlying medical conditions, others may occur during surgery itself and these often relate to anatomical or surgical access issues, and finally there are those that present postoperatively and which are often multifactorial in origin. Box 7.5 lists the post-laser surgery complications seen in a cohort of 82 of our patients treated by laser excision of oral precancer lesions or early invasive carcinomas over a 5-year period. The patients were followed up for 2 years post surgery [17].

In general, patients tolerate laser surgery extremely well, with only a minority reporting pain or postoperative bleeding and most of these are symptom-free within 2 months. Pain is not usually a major problem following laser treatment as vapourised wounds remain anaesthetic for several days, and standard analgesic regimes are usually sufficient to deal with discomfort.

Interestingly, and of considerable relevance to both patient information and education, is the observation that all of the post-treatment complications seen following laser surgery are most prevalent in those patients who continue to smoke and consume alcohol following surgery.

Reactionary haemorrhage in the hours following surgery is not uncommon but is usually minor and self-limiting. It is often associated with the use of aspirin or warfarin medication for pre-existing medical conditions or to the loss of vasoconstrictor effects as preoperatively administered local anaesthesia wears off. Nonetheless, it is prudent to admit most patients to hospital for observation the night following laser surgery, especially where large areas of mucosa have been excised.

Secondary haemorrhage occurring several days following laser can occur, usually following surgery to the tongue, and is predominantly due to superficial postoperative infection. Antibiotic therapy, topical mouthwashes with

---

Box 7.5 Complications following laser surgery

General and early effects
- Pain

- Swelling

- Bleeding

Site-specific effects
- Lingual nerve paraesthesia (lateral tongue)

- Obstructive submandibular sialadenitis (floor of mouth)

- Swallowing difficulties (soft palate and fauces)

- Speech difficulties (ventrolateral tongue)

Late effects
- Tongue tethering

- Recurrent disease

haemostatic agents such as tranexamic acid, rest and occasionally localised cauterisation of bleeding points are usually all that is required to deal with this complication. Rarely, patients may experience a severe post-surgical haemorrhage and surgical re-exploration may be required.

At some intra-oral sites, particularly the lateral tongue, localised irritation from adjacent dentition during the early stages of secondary intention healing may give rise to excessive granulation tissue forming localised, soft tissue swellings (Figure 7.29). Although sometimes quite alarming to patients, these lesions are easily recognised by their soft and mobile consistency and are easily excised under local anaesthesia either by scalpel or laser. It is best to send the excised tissue for histological examination to confirm the diagnosis and to exclude a neoplastic process.

Longer term post-surgery symptoms are predominantly related to anatomical complications. Tongue tethering, for example, may occur when ventrolateral lesions are excised and tongue tissue then becomes more tightly attached to the lingual mandibular alveolus during healing. Lingual nerve paraesthesia is seen most frequently following surgery to the lateral tongue, although this is usually a temporary phenomenon and most patients will have recovered by 1 year post surgery.

Submandibular salivary gland swelling due to ductal obstruction is not uncommon following anterior floor of mouth surgery. Due to the thin floor of mouth mucosa at this site, submandibular ducts are often involved during tissue dissection, although it is not usually necessary to formally explore or reposition damaged ducts as the majority of obstructive swellings settle spontaneously over time. In a small number of cases, gland obstruction may persist. These patients benefit from duct dilatation procedures, which may be carried out quite simply by inserting increasing diameters of lacrimal probes into the constricted duct to stretch the scarred tissue. Figure 7.30A illustrates post-laser floor of mouth scarring that can lead to constriction of the opening of the submandibular duct, whilst Figure 7.30B demonstrates the resultant submandibular salivary gland swelling due to such chronic obstructive sialadenitis. In Figure 7.30C a duct dilatation procedure is being undertaken. It is not known precisely at what time postoperatively duct dilatation should be carried out, but it is probably best done before 6 months to prevent permanent gland damage. Rarely, if gland symptoms persist, duct repositioning or formal submandibular gland removal may be required.

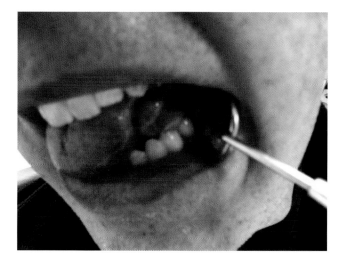

Figure 7.29 Exuberant granulation tissue may arise on the lateral tongue surface post laser, probably as a result of repetitive trauma from the adjacent teeth, as shown here. This usually heals rapidly following excision of the excess tissue.

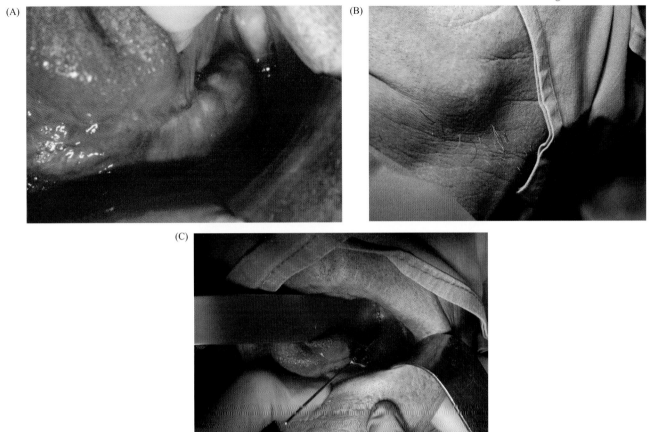

Figure 7.30 Following floor of mouth laser excision scarring may involve the submandibular duct (A) resulting in a chronic obstructive submandibular sialadenitis, which in rare cases may prove persistent (B), so that duct dilatation procedures using increasing diameters of lacrimal probes to stretch open the stricture may be necessary (C).

All general anaesthetic laser patients may experience a degree of sore throat in the immediate postoperative period due to the necessary endotracheal intubation with armoured tubes, but this usually resolves within a few days.

Long-term swallowing difficulties, whilst extremely unusual, tend to follow soft palate surgery. As with other intra-oral sites, excision is recommended but there is a small risk of oro-nasal fistula formation with large or deep excisions. Consequently, as we have previously discussed, if preoperative incisional biopsy has confirmed the presence of low-grade dysplasia only, then lesion ablation by de-focused laser vapourisation rather than excision may be an acceptable treatment.

Thermal damage and cytological artefacts may be seen histopathologically in CO_2 laser excision specimens and concerns have been raised in the past regarding potential difficulties in assessing damaged excision margins. However, these issues are well recognised by specialist oral pathologists and they are not usually a problem in practice nor does they seem to impair the ability to identify significant dysplasia in laser excision margins.

Laser surgical techniques have the considerable advantage of extending the treatment zone several millimetres beyond the excision specimen margins by adhering to the standard protocol of routine post-excision vapourisation of all wound margins. This has been described previously and is well demonstrated in the surgical cases above.

Combined treatment modalities

In oncology practice it is commonplace to combine therapeutic modalities to enhance treatment efficacy. For example, planned adjuvant postoperative radiotherapy or chemoradiotherapy is often administered following the surgical removal of head and neck tumours, especially extensive carcinomas exhibiting aggressive biological behaviour. However, combination treatments have rarely, if ever, been applied appropriately to the management of oral potentially malignant disorders. If we were able to identify those specific precancer patients who, following surgical excision, were at high risk of developing recurrent or further dysplastic disease or indeed of progressing to malignancy it would seem very logical and indeed highly desirable to try to coordinate additional medical or systemic therapies at the earliest stage of their treatment planning.

Whilst we will return to the problems inherent in trying to predict the clinical outcome of potentially malignant lesions in the next chapters of this book, the problem unfortunately remains that there is no good evidence at the present time to support the use of any individual or specific additional therapy.

This question may well, however, provide the basis for future randomised controlled clinical trials in oral precancer management and this would be welcomed. We will return to a more detailed discussion of future research methodologies and possible innovative treatment modalities in Chapter 10.

Patient follow up and surveillance

There are no clearly established guidelines for the follow up of treated oral precancer patients but all patients should certainly undergo a regular clinic review. It is best that this is tailored to individual patient disease profiling, rather than to arbitrary timetables. For example, during the first postoperative year it may be acceptable for patients whose lesions showed no or minimal dysplasia to be reviewed at 6-monthly intervals. However, 1-monthly follow-up appointments would seem to be much more appropriate for cases where severely dysplastic lesions had been excised.

Similarly, a patient who is no longer smoking, who has been able to address other risk factor behaviours such as reducing alcohol consumption, and who has recovered well from laser surgery with no overt clinical signs of residual mucosal disease may be seen less frequently than one who has not. It is important, therefore, to consciously determine a clinicopathological risk profile for each individual patient and to agree with them the precise detail and timing of their follow up.

There are also, unfortunately, no guidelines as to the overall length of time that patients should be followed up for, and by whom. Specialist oral precancer clinics may well follow up patients for several years, particularly those regarded as 'high-risk' cases, whilst other patients may be appropriately reviewed by primary care dental practitioners. In general, there is probably a consensus view that, similar to oral cancer patients, follow up for more severe dysplasia cases should be for at least 5 years since the last active phase of disease.

Indeed, continual reinforcement regarding risk factor behaviour at clinic follow-up appointments is very important. It encourages an overall surveillance management strategy that facilitates early diagnosis of recurrent or further disease and, most importantly, the identification of malignant transformation. Careful and thorough examination of all oral mucosal surfaces at each follow-up visit is important. It should be supplemented with diagnostic adjunctive techniques such as VELscope inspection and the use of brush biopsy sampling. All of these help to facilitate a truly active surveillance programme.

Indeed, it is now becoming increasingly recognised that surveillance within high-risk groups such as potentially malignant disorder patients is probably the only pragmatic and most realistic and efficacious manner of oral cancer and precancer screening [18].

Summary

The salient management goals in treating potentially malignant disorders have already been listed in Box 7.1 and, having now reviewed the currently available treatment options, it is possible for us to determine the effectiveness of each principal treatment modality in achieving these aims. The results are summarised in Table 7.2 and seem to support the view that surgical excision comes closest to being the optimal clinical management technique. Indeed, Mehanna et al. [19], following a recent systematic review and meta-analysis of published data on the management of oral dysplasia, commented that the only readily available and effective treatment for precancer is the surgical excision of individual lesions. This was felt likely to decrease the risk of malignant transformation of oral precancers by more than a half, but does not appear to eliminate the risk entirely [19].

Continued, active surveillance of patients following surgical excision of lesions therefore remains essential, especially for high-grade dysplasias, although the frequency and duration of the follow-up period should ideally be tailored to individual patient risk factors.

A flow chart is summarised in Figure 7.31 that demonstrates the recommended patient management strategy that we use in our oral dysplasia clinics in Newcastle. This is based upon the principle of interventional surgery and the complete excision and histopathological classification of identified precancer lesions. It illustrates how this can be applied to patients presenting with either single or multiple lesion disease.

We must now examine in some detail what actually happens to these patients following their interventional laser surgery, both in terms of their overall

Management goals	Treatment modality		
	Clinical observation	Medical treatment	Surgical excision
Accurate diagnosis	No	No	Yes
Early recognition of malignancy	Possibly	No	Yes
Removal of dysplastic mucosa	No	No	Yes
Prevention of recurrent or further disease	No	No	Possibly
Prevention of malignant transformation	No	No	Possibly
Minimal patient morbidity	Yes	No	Yes

Table 7.2 Effectiveness of oral precancer treatment modalities in achieving management goals.

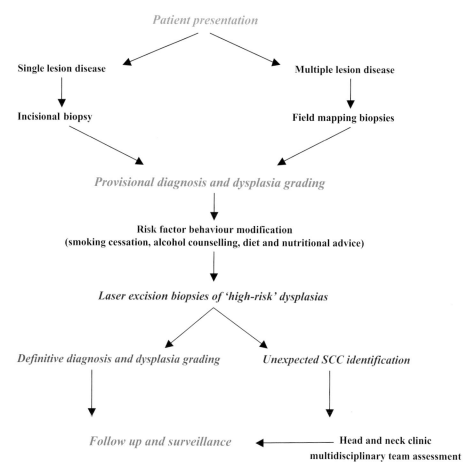

Figure 7.31 Interventional management strategy for oral precancer patients.

SCC, squamous cell carcinoma

clinical outcome and perhaps even more importantly their risk of developing oral squamous cell carcinoma. These issues will be addressed in the next two chapters of this book.

References

1. van der Waal I. Potentially malignant disorders of the oral and oropharyngeal mucosa; terminology, classification and present concepts of management. *Oral Oncol* 2009; 45: 317–323.
2. Thomson PJ, Wylie J. Interventional laser surgery: an effective surgical and diagnostic tool in oral precancer management. *Int J Oral Maxillofac Surg* 2002; 31: 145–153.
3. Goodson ML, Thomson PJ. Management of oral carcinoma – benefits of early precancerous intervention. *Br J Oral Maxillofac Surg* 2011; 49: 88–91.
4. Hamadah O, Hepburn S, Thomson PJ. Effects of active non-smoking programmes on smoking behaviour in oral precancer patients. *Int J Oral Maxillofac Surg* 2007; 36: 706–711.
5. Goodson ML, Hamadah O, Thomson PJ. The role of alcohol in oral precancer: observations from a North-East England population. *Br J Oral Maxillofac Surg* 2010; 48: 507–510.

6. Lancaster T, Stead L. Drug treatment for users of smokeless tobacco. *Br Med J* 2010; 341: 1228.
7. Thomson PJ, Goodson ML, Hamadah O. Cohort studies in oral precancer management: intervention vs. observation. *Oral Oncol* 2009; Suppl 3: 1 (abstract 116).
8. Lodi G, Sardella A, Bez C, Demarosi F, Carrassi A. Interventions for treating oral leukoplakia. *Cochrane Database Syst Rev* 2006; 4: CD001829.
9. Lodi G, Porter S. Management of potentially malignant disorders: evidence and critique. *J Oral Pathol Med* 2008; 37: 63–69.
10. Ribeiro AS, Salles PR, da Silva TA, Mesquita RA. A review of the nonsurgical treatment of oral leukoplakia. *Int J Dent* 2010; doi: 10.1155/2010/186018.
11. Marley JJ, Cowan CG, Linden GJ, Lamey PJ, Johnson NW, Warnakulasuriya KAAS. Management of potentially malignant oral mucosal lesions by consultant UK oral and maxillofacial surgeons. *Br J Oral Maxillofac Surg* 1996; 34: 28–36.
12. Marley JJ, Linden GJ, Cowan CG, Lamey PJ, Johnson NW, Warnakulasuriya KAAS, Scully C. A comparison of the management of potentially malignant oral mucosal lesions by oral medicine practitioners and oral and maxillofacial surgeons in the UK. *J Oral Pathol Med* 1998; 27: 489–495.
13. Stocker J, Thomson PJ, Hamadah O. Laser surgery in oral oncology – the Newcastle experience. *The Surgeon* 2005; Suppl 3: S32–33.
14. Hamadah O, Thomson PJ. Factors affecting carbon dioxide laser treatment for oral precancer: a patient cohort study. *Lasers Surg Med* 2009; 41: 17–25.
15. Hamadah O, Goodson ML, Thomson PJ. Clinicopathological behaviour of multiple oral dysplastic lesions compared with that of single lesions. *Br J Oral Maxillofac Surg* 2010; 48: 503–506.
16. Thomson PJ, Hamadah O. Cancerisation within the oral cavity: the use of 'field mapping biopsies' in clinical management. *Oral Oncol* 2007; 43: 20–26.
17. Goodson ML, Sugden K, Thomson PJ. Complications following interventional laser surgery for oral cancer and precancer. *Br J Oral Maxillofac Surg* 2011 (in press).
18. McGurk M, Scott SE. The reality of identifying early oral cancer in the general dental practice. *Br Dent J* 2010; 208: 347–351.
19. Mehanna HM, Rattay T, Smith J, McConkey CC. Treatment and follow-up of oral dysplasia – a systematic review and meta-analysis. *Head Neck* 2009; 31: 1600–1609.

8 Clinical Outcome

Peter Thomson

Oral Precancer: Diagnosis and Management of Potentially Malignant Disorders, First Edition. Edited by Peter Thomson.
© 2012 John Wiley & Sons, Ltd. Published 2012 by John Wiley & Sons, Ltd.

Introduction

Accurate, predictive assessment of the behaviour of oral precancers remains elusive in clinical practice. Yet establishing and defining clinical outcomes following the treatment of patients with potentially malignant disorders is absolutely fundamental to any discussion of management protocols. It is astonishing how little agreement exists in the literature on how such data should be analysed and discussed.

Clinical outcome may be defined overall as a measurement of how a patient feels, functions or indeed survives following disease recognition and treatment. Clearly, the most significant clinical outcome and the principal reason for identification and intervention in oral precancer is the prevention of malignant transformation and halting the development of oral cancer. This specific issue, however, will be explored and analysed in Chapter 9. In this chapter we will discuss in some detail the important overall clinical outcomes that may follow on from the diagnosis and treatment of oral potentially malignant disorders.

There are a number of difficulties inherent in trying to draw conclusions applicable to individual patient prognoses. These include:

- The lack of agreed terminology in published papers.

- The wide range of different types of lesions included in studies, particularly the analysis of non-dysplastic white patches, which unfortunately seems to confound the entire oral precancer literature.

- The varied treatment regimes and uncoordinated follow-up intervals involved.

Indeed, many studies in the literature are highly subjective and entirely retrospective in nature.

If one combines a range of study data obtained through the years, however, it is possible to make some very broad observations. In general, approximately 40% of dysplastic lesions probably change little or progress only slightly with time, whereas 20% may actually regress spontaneously. A further 20% will increase in size and extent, whilst the remaining 20% are at risk of progressing to malignancy. It must be emphasised that these are overall estimates based on population studies of both treated and non-treated lesions and, perhaps most significantly and very unhelpfully, do not in any way inform individual patient management.

Clinical outcome studies

It is surprisingly difficult to write definitively about the clinical outcome of oral precancer lesions because the available literature is so confusing in relation to terminology. There remains an enormous inconsistency between different authors and different studies. Similarly, the demonstrable lack of understanding of the natural history of oral potentially malignant disorders only confounds rather than clarifies our understanding.

What is also striking in reviewing published papers is the consensus observation that none of the perceived important and standard clinicopathological factors help to accurately predict clinical outcome [1]. Such factors include the clinical appearance of individual lesions, their anatomical site of origin, histopathological assessment, associated patient risk factor behaviour, and patient age or gender. Clinical outcome is itself, of course, influenced if not actually determined by the clinical management applied to individual cases. The fundamental problem with oral precancer remains the lack of internationally accepted treatment guidelines, a poor evidence base in the literature, and the paucity of relevant prospective, randomised clinical trials comparing different management strategies.

Many observational, anecdotal and retrospective papers have been published through the years. Unfortunately they add very little to our true understanding of the natural history and clinical outcome of oral potentially malignant disease, especially in relation to individual patient diagnosis and management. It is worth looking at two relatively recently published papers in detail because these illustrate quite well some of the inherent problems in trying to determine the true significance of clinical outcome for oral precancer patients.

Holmstrup et al. in 2006 reviewed long-term treatment outcomes for 269 premalignant lesions in 236 patients seen over a 20-year period [2]. One group of patients underwent surgical intervention and the other received no surgery. Histopathological data and risk of malignant transformation were reported for 94 surgically excised lesions and compared with 175 non-surgically treated lesions. However, as a retrospective review, the authors admit that they are unable to explain how treatment decisions were made for all of their reported cases. They stated that 12% of surgically treated lesions developed carcinoma after a mean follow-up period of 7.5 years, compared with only 4% of non-surgically treated lesions after a mean of 6.6 years follow up. It is important to appreciate, however, that the two groups were actually non-comparable. Whilst 71% of the surgically excised lesions were dysplastic and often severely so, only 12% of the non-surgically treated lesions displayed any dysplasia whatsoever and if present it was usually categorised as mild.

This is one of the commonest and most persistent difficulties found in the literature when one attempts to interpret the true relevance of clinical outcome papers. If many cases are included in analyses that have never shown dysplasia on biopsy, comparison of outcome with dysplasia patients is probably entirely meaningless. So that, despite the large number of patients included and the availability of follow-up data for up to 20 years (although the mean was actually only between 5.5 years for non-surgical and 6.8 years for surgical cases), Holmstrup's series is a non-randomised retrospective review with effectively non-comparable groups. This renders the results of questionable or perhaps even no true biological significance.

Arduino et al. in 2009, similarly, retrospectively reviewed the outcome of 207 oral dysplastic lesions treated over a 16-year period by a variety of surgical excisions, cryotherapies or clinical observation alone [1]. They noted that over a median 4.5-year follow-up period, 39% lesions disappeared, 20% remained stable, 34% developed new dysplastic lesions and 7% developed a squamous cell carcinoma [1]. Whilst the authors of this paper found no significant differences in outcome between treated and untreated lesions, the study group was so heterogeneous and patient data collected over such a long study period that once again the results must be interpreted with real caution.

The limitations of the above non-randomised patient studies are obvious and the potential for clinician bias in treatment selection, however well meaning, severely limits scientific validity and clinical relevance. Interestingly, both the above papers share the same unsurprising conclusion that randomised controlled clinical trials are advised because of the inherent weaknesses of such retrospective reviews.

Patient cohort studies

It is probably true to say that, whilst there is no strictly universally agreed hierarchy of biomedical evidence, randomised controlled trials rank much higher in terms of scientific methodology than observational studies, expert opinion and anecdotal experience. Many authors would also now add that systematic reviews and meta-analyses should rank even higher than controlled trials as they combine data from a variety of different studies and sources.

Randomised controlled trials are favoured because they probably best eliminate investigator bias and potential confounding factors by randomly assigning patients to one type of intervention or another, or indeed often to a non-intervention or placebo arm. Whilst this may be scientifically valid, such trials are not always appropriate or acceptable to patients or clinicians in the medical environment. As we have seen in Chapter 7, there have been attempts to design randomised trials for oral precancer medical treatments but these have largely proved unsuccessful, unreliable and have produced little of clinical relevance.

Many authors, as exampled above, correctly bemoan the lack of meaningful randomised trials for oral precancer management. However, there are clinical difficulties in randomising potentially malignant disease patients, especially to non-treatment study arms, when there remains such an unpredictable and biologically devastating risk of malignant transformation.

Cohort studies, on the other hand, do offer opportunities for longitudinal observational analysis of a group of people who share either a common characteristic or experience within a defined time period. There are a number of potential advantages to patient cohort studies in oral precancer research and these are summarised in Box 8.1. The longitudinal observation of a group of patients through time and the collection of data at regular intervals can actually produce data superior to those of cross-sectional and retrospective studies. Indeed, this is often the recommended methodology in observational epidemiology.

In the absence of multicentre, randomised, prospective clinical trials we will describe in this chapter the results of a series of patient cohort studies carried out in our dysplasia clinics in Newcastle upon Tyne in northern England. Whilst not

---

Box 8.1 Advantages of oral precancer patient cohort studies.

- Defined study population sharing common characteristics and risk factor behaviour

- Inclusion criteria facilitate recruitment of cases with proven dysplasia

- Standard diagnostic procedures

- Agreed treatment protocol and standardised intervention

- Consistent clinical decision making

- Longitudinal observation of subjects with documented clinical follow up

> **Box 8.2** Definitions of clinical outcome.
>
> - *Clinical resolution*: Patient is clinically free of oral precancer disease
> - *Persistent disease*: Oral precancer lesion persists clinically despite interventional treatment
> - *Recurrent disease*: Oral precancer lesion recurs at same site following previous excision
> - *Further disease*: New-site development of oral precancer lesion(s)
> - *Malignant transformation*: Oral squamous cell carcinoma arising at the site of a clinically recognised precursor lesion
> - *Oral cancer development*: Oral squamous cell carcinoma developing at a new site distant from precursor lesions

necessarily universally applicable, these studies benefit from a defined and static patient population known to be at high risk of oral cancer, a consistent and coordinated clinical management protocol coordinated by one clinician, and a regular and consistent follow-up strategy, as outlined in Chapter 7.

Definitions of clinical outcome

It is important at the outset, before describing and attempting to analyse our patient cohort data, to define the parameters by which the clinical outcome and evolution of precancer disease should be assessed. As we have seen, the literature in this field is full of so many differing terminologies that meta-analysis is rendered extremely complicated, if not actually impossible. We recommend the following terms, which are summarised in Box 8.2. They are firmly based upon several observational studies we have carried out on cohorts of new patients presenting with dysplastic oral precancer lesions who have been carefully followed up subsequent to interventional laser surgery. The categories of malignant transformation and development of oral squamous cell carcinoma, however, will be discussed in Chapter 9.

Clinical resolution (disease-free state)

Clinical resolution is the successful surgical removal or regression of a potentially malignant disorder resulting in clinically normal-looking oral mucosa with no further precancer lesion arising either at the site of previous disease or elsewhere in the oral cavity or oropharynx.

An example of clinical resolution following laser excision of a lateral tongue precancer lesion is shown in Figure 8.1. Figure 8.2 also illustrates an example of clinical resolution, although in this case floor of mouth scarring has created a white appearance which may be mistaken for persistent or recurrent leukoplakia. Such scarring may also give rise to confusion under VELscope® examination, where scar tissue can appear dark on tissue autofluorescence due to the increased vasculature in the immediately subjacent tissue.

Overall, in our studies we have observed that 76% of laser-treated patients may be disease-free 18 months after surgery, although this falls with increased length of follow-up periods, dropping to around 64% by 5 years. Thus, the

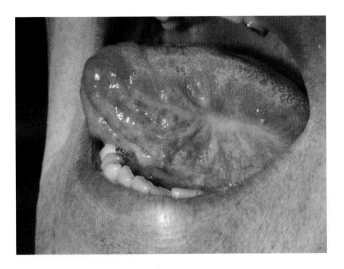

Figure 8.1 Clinical resolution following laser excision of a dysplastic leukoplakia from the lateral surface of the tongue. Two years post laser there is no evidence of further precancer disease at this site.

longer patients are followed up, the more chance there is of identifying new potentially malignant disease development and this is a very important observation for clinical management strategies.

Persistent disease

Persistent disease is the term used to describe potentially malignant lesions that persist at the same site following treatment. Thus, once postoperative healing has stabilised and despite whole lesion excision, there is evidence of a residual precancer lesion which can be seen and identified clinically.

Such persistent lesions usually have an identical clinical appearance and exhibit the same histopathological features as their original presenting lesion. A clinical example of persistent leukoplakia following laser excision of a soft palate lesion is shown in Figure 8.3.

In our experience, persistence of precancer disease is a relatively rare occurrence. Whilst there are no clear factors to explain why it occurs, it is possible that technical limitations during surgery may leave dysplastic tissue in situ. It is also possible that microscopically changed and genetically primed, but clinically normal-looking, mucosa is 'activated' to progress to a clinically observable lesion following surgery. There is no doubt, however, that persistent disease is more common when, for the reasons outlined in Chapter 7, laser ablation has been performed instead of formal laser excision of whole lesions.

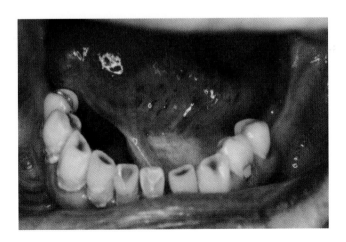

Figure 8.2 Clinical resolution following floor of mouth laser excision at 1 year postoperatively. Note the pale scar tissue which on superficial inspection may resemble leukoplakia.

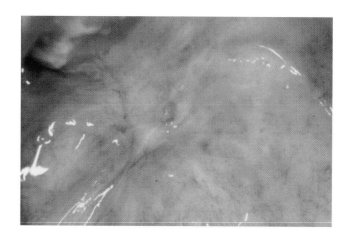

Figure 8.3 An example of persistent disease, illustrating an erosive leukoplakia at the site of a recent soft palate laser excision.

Recurrent disease (same-site recurrence)

Recurrent disease is the term used to describe lesions that reappear at the same site following a treatment which had apparently brought about clinical resolution for a time.

We have found it to affect approximately 16% of our patients after laser surgery and have identified persistent tobacco smoking and alcohol as significant risk factors for disease to recur in this manner. Whilst the precise time to clinical recurrence varies, it is most common to see recurrent lesions during the first 2 years of patient follow up. Such recurrent disease usually presents with the same clinical appearance of the previously treated lesion and arises at the same site, as illustrated on the lateral tongue in Figure 8.4.

It may be difficult to distinguish recurrent lesions from post-laser scar tissue initially (see Figure 8.2), although as patients are under regular review careful clinical examination should identify changes in mucosal appearance. It may be helpful in these situations to utilise adjunctive diagnostic techniques, such as tissue autofluorescence, to visualise potentially abnormal mucosa at an early stage. Again, the presence of scar tissue can make the appearance more difficult to interpret.

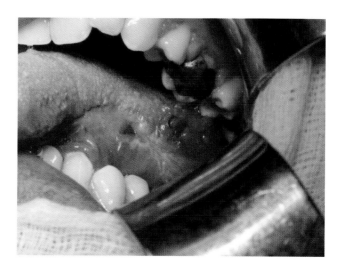

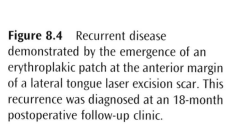

Figure 8.4 Recurrent disease demonstrated by the emergence of an erythroplakic patch at the anterior margin of a lateral tongue laser excision scar. This recurrence was diagnosed at an 18-month postoperative follow-up clinic.

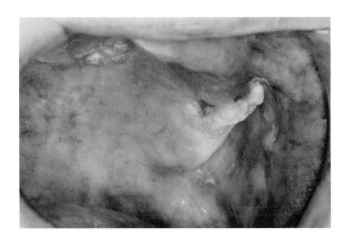

Figure 8.5 Further disease in a patient developing multiple verrucous leukoplakic lesions bilaterally in the maxillary alveolus and palatal mucosa following previous successful excision of a buccal mucosa leukoplakia.

Further disease (new-site recurrence)

Further disease is defined as the development of additional precancer lesions at new, distinct sites in the oral cavity, which appear after successful treatment of pre-existing lesions.

This occurs in about 14% of patients following laser excision and is an important clinical manifestation of field cancerisation, demonstrating the inherent instability of oral mucosa in potentially malignant disorder patients. Figure 8.5 shows a clinical example of further disease, appearing in this case as multiple verrucous leukoplakic lesions in the maxillary alveolar and palatal mucosa, approximately 12 months following successful laser excision of a buccal leukoplakia.

Patients who continue to smoke and consume alcohol are again at particular risk of further disease, although interestingly we have also observed a high risk of further lesion development in non-smokers and non-alcohol consumers. This latter observation probably results from an inherently unstable oral mucosa in the absence of identifiable aetiological agents. Indeed, we have also observed the presence of larger and more severely dysplastic precancer lesions in non-smoking patients compared with smokers.

Newcastle patient cohort studies

At this juncture it would seem useful to review and explore in some detail the various clinical outcomes we have documented in a series of longitudinal patient cohort studies carried out in our dysplasia clinics in Newcastle upon Tyne over the last 15 years. In all of the studies referred to below the patients' ages and gender were consistent, with a male patient predominance and a mean age of around 60 years, and with the vast majority being regular tobacco and alcohol users. Most of the clinical lesions treated were leukoplakias arising in the floor of the mouth and ventral tongue, which primarily exhibited moderate to severe dysplasia histopathologically.

In the following interventional laser studies standardised treatment protocols, as described in Chapter 7, were commenced following preoperative evaluation, incisional biopsy to determine a provisional dysplasia diagnosis, and laser excision of lesions. These stages were all carried out within 6–8 weeks of the initial biopsy by the same surgeon.

Interventional laser study 1 (Thomson & Wylie 2002)

In this study, 57 consecutive patients presenting over a 4-year period (1996 to 2000) and undergoing laser excision of 55 dysplastic precancer lesions were followed for a mean period of 18 months and their clinical outcome documented. Of these cases, 76% remained disease-free following laser treatment, whilst 6% developed recurrent disease and 12% went on to exhibit further precancer disease. Malignant transformation and cancer development occurred in 6% of cases overall [3].

Interventional laser study 2 (Stocker et al. 2005)

The results of 199 patients undergoing laser surgery for 248 precancer lesions over a 7-year period (1997 to 2004) were reviewed. We found that overall 67% of patients remained disease-free, with 15% experiencing recurrent disease and 14% developing further disease at new intra-oral sites, mostly within 2 years of initial diagnosis. There were no instances of same-site malignant transformation but in 4% of cases oral carcinoma developed at new sites [4].

Interventional laser study 3 (Thomson et al. 2008)

This investigation followed 40 new patients presenting with single dysplastic lesions treated by laser excision and followed for 5 years post treatment. We observed that 60% of patients were disease-free at 5 years, whereas 22% suffered same-site recurrence and 18% went on to develop further disease at new sites. There were no instances of malignancy in this study group [5].

Interventional laser study 4 (Hamadah & Thomson 2009)

Seventy-eight consecutive, new, single precancer lesion patients were followed for a mean period of 5 years following interventional laser surgery. Overall, 64% of patients remained disease-free, although interestingly detailed analysis showed a drop from an 86% disease-free survival at 2 years post surgery to 69% at 5 years. Eighteen percent of patients developed recurrence and 14% further disease, whilst 4% of patients developed an oral carcinoma, but all of these occurred at sites distant from their initial precancer lesions [6,7].

Of specific interest in this case series were the observations that neither the definitive histopathological diagnosis of the excised lesion nor the presence of dysplasia in excision margins significantly influenced clinical outcome. Smokers, however, appeared to be at higher risk of developing recurrence of their dysplastic lesions [6,7].

Observational study (Goodson et al. 2008)

In order to investigate the effectiveness of observational management, a small cohort of 30 new patients presenting with single oral precancer lesions, showing either mild or moderate dysplasia, were followed for a mean of 4 years post diagnosis. The patients were treated conservatively by clinical observation and risk factor modification alone (without laser surgery) [8].

In 25 cases we found that clinical lesions persisted unchanged, which is probably not surprising, although five resolved completely and one demonstrated some clinical improvement. There were no instances of malignancy development in this cohort. Whilst five patients reduced their smoking, only two actually stopped smoking completely during the follow-up period and these behavioural changes did not significantly affect the observed clinical outcome.

Repeat incisional biopsies were carried out on the 25 persistent lesions, at a mean interval of 2.8 years, and demonstrated no change in histopathological diagnosis in just over half of the biopsies. In the remaining ten cases, however, there was some apparent improvement in histological diagnoses with initially mildly dysplastic grades subsequently reported as hyperkeratoses, and moderate dysplasia becoming mild. Of course, as lesions remained unexcised, such 'improvements' might actually be a reflection of sampling errors during biopsies.

Clearly, this study population is limited by clinician selection bias but nonetheless is an interesting patient group from the same geographical location and of similar age and gender to our laser surgery cohorts [8].

Intervention versus observation study (Thomson et al. 2009)

In this investigation we wished to make a direct comparison between treated and non-treated groups, and as outlined in the previous chapter, we undertook a further cohort study. In this study, following incisional biopsy diagnosis of dysplasia, the outcomes for 78 patients who underwent laser excision of a precancer lesions were compared with a group of 39 patients who were managed conservatively by clinical observation alone [9].

Interestingly, 84% of laser-treated patients who were designated 'high risk' and who had primarily severe and moderately dysplastic lesions remained disease-free for 3 years following treatment. However, only 23% of observed lesions that were mainly mildly dysplastic or 'low risk' in nature showed any clinical resolution [9].

The Newcastle 10-year follow-up study (Diajil 2011)

Most recently, Diajil has studied in considerable detail long-term clinical outcomes for a cohort of 100 single dysplastic lesion patients treated in Newcastle by interventional laser surgical excision. This is probably the most important data set studied to date as it exams a cohort of patients managed by one clinical team, working to agreed treatment protocols and with up to 10 years documented follow up [10].

In general, Diajil found that at their most recent follow-up appointments, 62% of patients were completely disease-free following laser surgery, 17% had developed recurrent (same-site) disease, whilst 14% experienced further (new-site) disease. Five percent of potentially malignant disorders in this cohort underwent same-site malignant transformation, with another 2% developing an oral squamous cell carcinoma at a site distinct from their original precancer lesion. We will discuss the issue of malignancy in more detail in the next chapter, however.

Thus, our overall clinical outcome data now appear remarkably consistent across a number of specific longitudinal patient cohort studies and these are summarised in Table 8.1 for comparison. Overall we can predict that 66% of our patients are likely to remain disease-free following laser surgery, with 16%

Clinical outcome/ study features	Study				
	Thomson & Wylie (2002)	Stocker et al. (2005)	Thomson et al. (2008)	Hamadah & Thomson (2009)	Diajil (2011)
Clinical resolution	76%	67%	60%	64%	62%
Recurrent disease	6%	15%	22%	18%	18%
Further disease	12%	14%	18%	14%	14%
Malignant transformation	4%	0%	0%	0%	5%
OSCC development	2%	4%	0%	4%	2%
No. of patients	57	199	40	78	100
Study period (years)	4	7	5	10	10
Mean follow up (years)	1.5	NR	5	5	10

OSCC, oral squamous cell carcinoma; NR, not reported.

Table 8.1 Clinical outcome data for interventional laser surgery (Newcastle cohort studies).

at risk of recurrent disease and 14% at risk of further precancers arising at new sites. The overall risk for same-site malignant transformation and cancer development at a new oral site remains low at approximately 4%.

Diajil, however, further analysed clinical outcome in relation to the length of follow up and by plotting precancer disease-free survival via Kaplan–Meier survival analysis showed a clear relationship with time (Figure 8.6). Whilst 88% of patients were disease-free at 1 year post surgery there was a progressive rise in recurrent and further disease observed through successive years so that at 10 years post laser only 42% of patients remained free of dysplastic disease. This is a highly significant observation and extremely important for patient follow up.

As illustrated in more detail in Figure 8.7, recurrence of a precancer lesion (same site) is most likely to occur within the first 2 years following laser surgery. Such patients tend to be older and usually present initially with larger lesions showing more significant dysplastic change.

In contradistinction to recurrence, further disease (new-site presentation) can arise at any time within the first 5 years of follow up, as demonstrated in Figure 8.8. This, of course, reflects widespread field cancerisation within the oral cavity and as we have already discussed is a significant clinical management

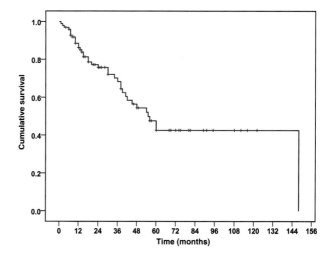

Figure 8.6 Overall disease-free survival following potentially malignant lesion excision, as plotted by Kaplan–Meier analysis. There is a steady fall in disease-free status over time so that whilst 88% of patients showed clinical resolution at 1 year post surgery, this fell to 42% by 10 years (Diajil 2011 [10]).

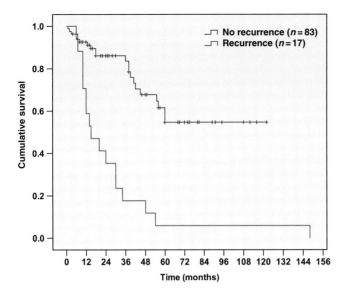

Figure 8.7 Kaplan–Meier survival analysis confirms that the onset of recurrent disease (same-site recurrence) is most commonly seen within the first 2 years following laser surgery excision (Diajil 2011 [10]).

problem for these patients, particularly as few consistent features appear to help predict such outcome.

Interestingly, on reclassifying excised lesions utilising the binary (high/low grade) dysplasia classification system discussed in Chapter 6, Diajil demonstrated a significant risk of lower overall disease-free status for those lesions identified as 'high grade'. The Kaplan–Meier analysis for this is illustrated in Figure 8.9.

In relation to patients who present with multiple precancer lesions, reporting and analysis of follow-up data is much more difficult because it is confounded by the widespread nature of pre-existing mucosal disease at various intra-oral sites. Assessments of the categories of persistent or further disease are especially problematic in this regard [11].

Patient follow up

Through the years many clinicians and observers have noted, particularly in relation to head and neck cancer, the limited efficacy of patient follow-up clinics in identifying recurrent disease and second primary tumours. Indeed, it is often the patients themselves that alert clinicians to suspicious signs and symptoms when they re-attend clinics. There is no doubt, however, in relation to oral potentially malignant disease that a coordinated and detailed follow up,

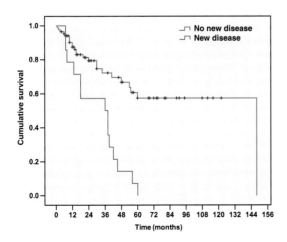

Figure 8.8 Kaplan–Meier survival analysis shows that the onset of further disease (new-site disease) may occur at any time during the first 5 years of follow up (Diajil 2011 [10]).

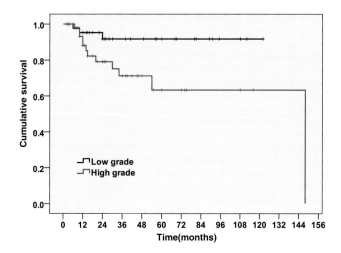

Figure 8.9 Applying the binary dysplasia grading system to excised precancer lesions, Kaplan–Meier analysis demonstrates a significantly higher risk of recurrent and further disease presentation at 2 and 5 years post surgery for high-grade dysplasias (log rank test $P = 0.013$) (Diajil 2011 [10]).

supplemented by diagnostic adjuncts to visualise and inspect oral mucosa in detail, does indeed help to identify recurrent or further disease at the earliest possible stage, alongside the important opportunities to identify the presence of early malignant change. It is vital that the clinician carries out a comprehensive oral cavity examination at each review appointment, in view of the recognition of field change cancerisation and the likelihood of both further precancer disease and also carcinoma development especially arising at new intra-oral sites.

Follow up is thus recognised as fundamental and integral to complete and satisfactory patient care and the principle of active surveillance is as important as any other aspect of an interventional management protocol. We know that patients who continue to smoke and drink alcohol are at particular risk of recurrent disease following laser surgery and a more rigorous clinic follow-up schedule is probably appropriate for these cases [7,12].

It must also be remembered, of course, that younger non-smoking patients with no other discernable risk factor behaviour may also be at high risk of further disease and malignant transformation [13].

Prediction of clinical outcome

Accurate prediction of the behaviour of oral potentially malignant disorders remains a problem in modern clinical practice. Development of management strategies in the future will require robust predictive techniques to identify individual patients and lesions at risk of poor clinical outcome and cancer development.

Although still very much in the research stage, it is both interesting and informative regarding the natural history of potentially malignant disorders to review the results of studies carried out to investigate the potential role of predictive tools in determining clinical outcome following precancer treatment.

As we have seen in Chapter 3, increasing dysregulation of epithelial cell proliferation is fundamental to carcinogenesis and such features may be characterised and studied in epithelial tissue via immunohistochemical analyses. These techniques were introduced in Chapter 2 in relation to the study of normal oral mucosal structure and function. Interestingly, in preliminary studies that we carried out some years ago we confirmed the presence of increased cell proliferative labelling indices in oral tissue specimens demonstrating increasing levels of dysplasia [14]. These data are summarised diagrammatically in Figure 8.10.

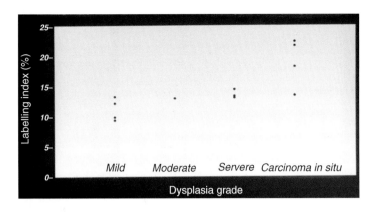

Figure 8.10 Cell proliferative labelling indices plotted against dysplasia grading for a series of 12 precancer lesions, showing a 2.3% increase in labelling with each increasing grade of dysplasia (*P* = 0.01) *(Reproduced from Thomson et al. 1999 [14], with permission from Elsevier).*

We also subsequently discovered demonstrable changes in proliferative activity with enhanced suprabasal labelling as epithelial tissue becomes increasingly disorganised and dysplasia extends through the higher epithelial layers [15]. These features are shown histopathologically in Figure 8.11 for cyclin A labelling, and are summarised in graphic representation in Figure 8.12 using Ki67 labelling as an overall marker of cell proliferative activity.

More recently we have used computer-assisted microscope systems to produce quantitative and highly reproducible analyses of proliferative cell activity. These techniques can be applied to archived paraffin-embedded tissue specimens previously excised from precancer patients. Combining the histopathological diagnoses with quantitative proliferative labelling indices and documented patient clinical outcome following laser treatment provides a unique way to investigate a possible predictive tool [5,16].

In a study re-analysing tissue specimens from 40 patients treated by laser excision and followed for 5 years postoperatively, cell cyclin markers A and B1, together with the proliferative marker Ki67, were assessed as predictors of clinical outcome. Both cyclin A (a cycle protein produced during the S phase and required to help drive cells through S into G2 and then mitosis) and cyclin B1 (which primarily measures the G2 to mitosis transition), together with Ki67 (which is an overall marker of proliferative activity), showed increased expression with worsening dysplasia through mild, moderate and severe categories [5]. The increased cell proliferative activity is graphically represented in Figure 8.13, whilst Figures 8.14–8.16 illustrate the appearance of immunohistochemically labelled dysplastic specimens using cyclin A, cyclin B1 and Ki67 respectively.

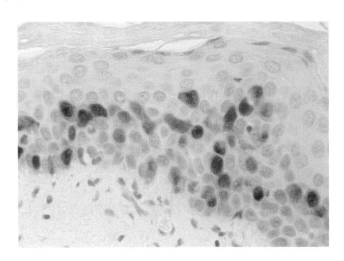

Figure 8.11 Immunohistochemical labelling showing cyclin A activity extending to the suprabasal layers in a moderate dysplasia tissue specimen.

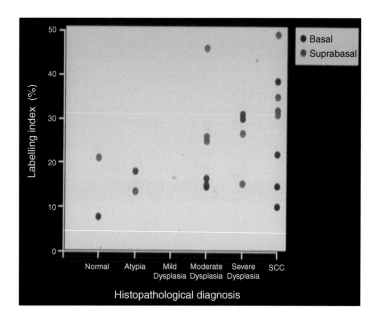

Figure 8.12 Plot of basal cell and suprabasal cell Ki67 labelling in 11 excised precancer and cancer lesions. Note the predominance of high suprabasal labelling in the severe dysplasia and carcinoma categories. SCC, squamous cell carcinoma. *(Reproduced from Thomson et al. 2002 [15].)*

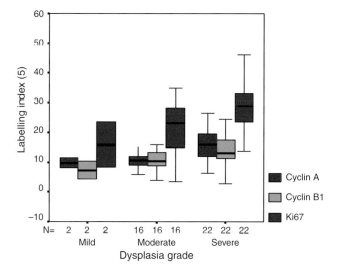

Figure 8.13 Increasing labelling indices for cyclin A and B1 and Ki67 seen with increasing grades of dysplasia in 40 laser excised precancer specimens *(Reproduced from Thomson et al. 2008 [5], with permission from Elsevier).*

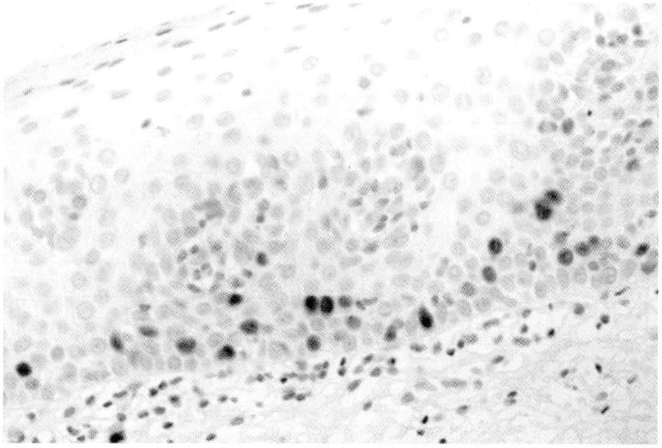

Figure 8.14 Immunohistochemical identification of cyclin A labelling in a moderately dysplastic tissue specimen.

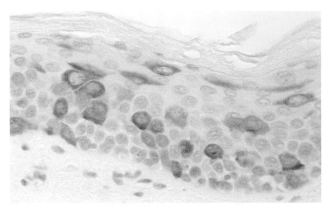

Figure 8.15 Immunohistochemical identification of cyclin B1 labelling in an atrophic, severely dysplastic epithelial sample.

Of particular interest were the results seen when Kaplan–Meier disease-free survival analyses were carried out for these cases, using the onset of recurrent or further disease as step function. Median labelling indices were used as cut-off points for cyclin A (12%), cyclin B1 (12%) and Ki67 (22%) demonstrating a significantly higher incidence of disease recurrence in lesions exhibiting higher proliferative labelling indices (Figures 8.17–8.19) [5].

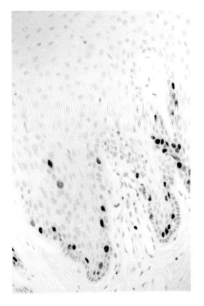

Figure 8.16 Immunohistochemical identification of Ki67 labelling, predominantly in the basal layers, in a mild dysplasia specimen.

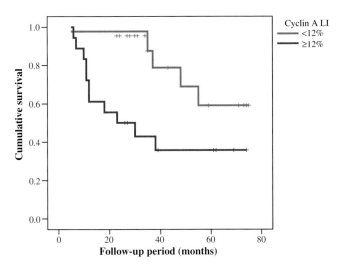

Figure 8.17 Kaplan–Meier plot of cyclin A labelling indices (LI) demonstrating significantly reduced disease-free survival when labelling is higher than the median value of 12% (log rank chi-square, $P = 0.01$) *(Reproduced from Thomson et al. 2008 [5], with permission from Elsevier).*

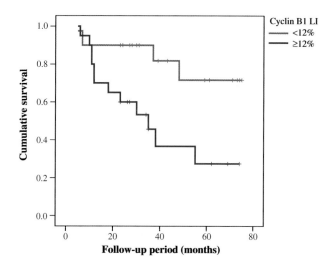

Figure 8.18 Kaplan–Meier plot of cyclin B1 labelling indices (LI) demonstrating significantly reduced disease-free survival when labelling is higher than the median value of 12% (log rank chi-square, $P = 0.01$) (Reproduced from Thomson et al 2008 [5], with permission from Elsevier).

Thus, we appear to have a quantitative measure of cell proliferative activity that correlates well to increasing severity of dysplasia seen in potentially malignant lesions and which can be significantly linked to worsening clinical outcome. In addition, such immunohistochemical techniques preserve both the epithelial structure and the important relationship between epithelium and the underlying connective tissue.

The importance of the epithelial tissue structure and the resulting disruption seen in dysplasia were illustrated in studies in which we demonstrated significant proliferative variations in the epithelial hierarchical organisation. We found that enhanced suprabasal cyclin A activity – which is essentially a visual demonstration of increased cell proliferative activity, encompassing larger growth fractions and shortened cell cycle times within tissue – was also associated with poor clinical outcome in terms of persistent or further precancer disease development [15].

As yet, such epithelial proliferative studies are primarily research tools. It remains uncertain whether the identification of patients and individual potentially malignant lesions with predicted poor clinical outcome will ultimately alter disease progression. It is, however, not an unreasonable hypothesis that an early identification of such cases might rationalise therapeutic intervention, marshall systemic therapies and, as discussed in Chapter 7, may allow the coordination of combined modality treatment at the earliest stages of clinical management.

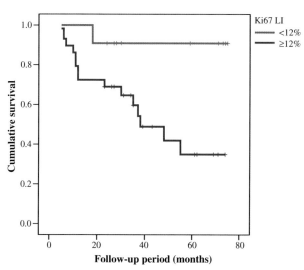

Figure 8.19 Kaplan–Meier plot of Ki67 labelling indices (LI) demonstrating significantly reduced disease-free survival when labelling is higher than the median value of 22% (log rank chi-square, $P = 0.03$) (Reproduced from Thomson et al. 2008 [5], with permission from Elsevier).

Summary

The ability to predict or even to determine defined clinical outcomes for potentially malignant disorders remains elusive in clinical practice. This is partly due to a lack of understanding of the natural history of the disease, confusion over terminology, limited agreement on therapeutic interventions and uncertainty regarding patient follow up. Defining the parameters by which outcome may be measured and the longitudinal study of patient cohorts undergoing treatment probably offer the best opportunities to increase our knowledge of oral precancer disease. Ultimately, the goal of potentially malignant lesion diagnosis and treatment is the prevention of squamous cell carcinoma. It is this crucially important and potentially devastating outcome that we will consider in detail in Chapter 9.

References

1. Arduino PG, Surace A, Carbone M, Elia A, Massolini G, Gandolfo S, Broccoletti R. Outcome of oral dysplasia: a retrospective hospital-based study of 207 patients with a long follow up. *J Oral Pathol Med* 2009; 38: 540–544.
2. Holmstrup P, Vedtofte P, Reibel J, Stoltze K. Long-term treatment outcome of oral premalignant lesions. *Oral Oncol* 2006; 42: 461–474.
3. Thomson PJ, Wylie J. Interventional laser surgery: an effective surgical and diagnostic tool in oral precancer management. *Int J Oral Maxillofac Surg* 2002; 31: 145–153.
4. Stocker J, Thomson PJ, Hamadah O. Laser surgery in oral oncology – the Newcastle experience. *The Surgeon* 2005; Suppl 3: S32–33.
5. Thomson PJ, Hamadah O, Goodson ML, Cragg N, Booth C. Predicting recurrence after oral precancer treatment: use of cell cycle analysis. *Br J Oral Maxillofac Surg* 2008; 46: 370–375.
6. Hamadah O, Thomson PJ. Factors affecting carbon dioxide laser treatment for oral precancer: a patient cohort study. *Laser Surg Med* 2009; 41: 17–25.
7. Hamadah O, Hepburn S, Thomson PJ. Effects of active non-smoking programmes on smoking behaviour in oral precancer patients. *Int J Oral Maxillofac Surg* 2007; 36: 706–711.
8. Goodson ML, Hamadah O, Thomson PJ. Conservative management of oral precancer: outcomes for a north-east cohort. *Presentation, PanEuropean Federation, International Association of Dental Research*, London, 2008.
9. Thomson PJ, Goodson ML, Hamadah O. Cohort studies in oral precancer management: intervention vs. observation. *Oral Oncol* 2009; 3 (Suppl 1): 116
10. Diajil A. Personal communication, 2011.
11. Hamadah O, Goodson ML, Thomson PJ. Clinicopathological behaviour of multiple oral dysplastic lesions compared with that of single lesions. *Br J Oral Maxillofac Surg* 2010; 48: 503–506.
12. Goodson ML, Hamadah O, Thomson PJ. The role of alcohol in oral precancer: observations from a north-east population. *Br J Oral Maxillofac Surg* 2010; 48: 507–510.
13. Diajil A, Goodson ML, Thomson PJ. Smoking behaviour and oral potentially malignant disorders – bad news for non-smokers. *15th International Congress on Oral Pathology and Medicine Abstract Book*, 2010: 136.
14. Thomson PJ, Potten CS, Appleton DR. Characterization of epithelial cell activity in patients with oral cancer. *Br J Oral Maxillofac Surg* 1999; 37: 384–390.
15. Thomson PJ, Soames JV, Booth C, O'Shea JA. Epithelial cell proliferative activity and oral cancer progression. *Cell Proliferat* 2002; 35 (Suppl 1): 110–120.
16. Thomson PJ, Goodson ML, Booth C, Cragg N, Hamadah O. Cyclin A activity predicts clinical outcome in oral precancer and cancer. *Int J Oral Maxillofac Surg* 2006; 35: 1041–1046.

9 Malignant Transformation and Oral Cancer Development

Peter Thomson

Oral Precancer: Diagnosis and Management of Potentially Malignant Disorders, First Edition. Edited by Peter Thomson.
© 2012 John Wiley & Sons, Ltd. Published 2012 by John Wiley & Sons, Ltd.

Introduction

The transformation of precursor potentially malignant lesions into invasive carcinoma must be seen as the ultimate failure in diagnosis and management of oral precancer. Clinical examples of squamous cell carcinoma that have arisen from pre-existing tongue leukoplakias are illustrated in Figures 9.1 and 9.2. The fact that such oral leukoplakias still unpredictably transform into cancers remains a major frustration to clinicians, particularly as we are still unable to predict how quickly or how likely any individual patient or any potentially malignant disorder will proceed towards cancerisation.

Quoted transformation rates to oral malignancy vary widely in the published literature, from around 0.1% to over 40%. The interpretation of such data is complicated by the heterogeneous clinical and histopathological nature of different precursor lesions studied and the varying length of follow-up periods in different reported series.

In Chapter 8 we considered the overall spectrum of clinical outcomes that may be seen following the diagnosis and management of oral precancer lesions. Unfortunately, many of the difficulties we experienced in interpreting the available scientific literature to enhance our understanding of the natural history of the disease apply equally well to our desire to clarify our knowledge of oral carcinogenesis. In this chapter, therefore, we will review some of the salient concepts surrounding our current understanding of oral precancer transformation to malignancy and, using data obtained from observational studies following cohorts of treated Newcastle patients (see Chapter 8), will

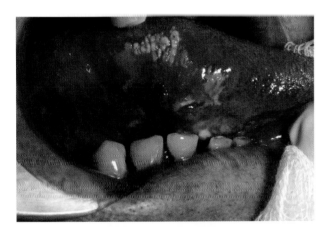

Figure 9.1 An infiltrative squamous cell carcinoma arising in a pre-existing non-homogeneous leukoplakia on the ventrolateral tongue.

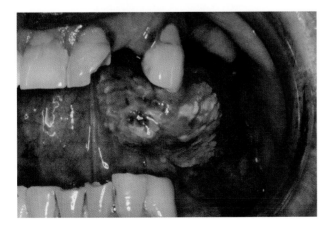

Figure 9.2 An ulcerative squamous cell carcinoma arising from a pre-existing non-homogeneous ventral tongue leukoplakia.

make recommendations both for the terminology of disease recognition and for clinical patient management.

Risk of progression to oral carcinoma

There are, unfortunately, very few reliable data sets available in the literature that help to provide either a consensus or a pragmatic view regarding the risk of cancer development in oral potentially malignant disorder patients. Figure 9.3 summarises the clinical dilemma in predicting the likely clinical outcome in a patient who presented with widespread, multiple foci of ventral tongue and floor of mouth leukoplakia.

An overall malignant transformation rate of approximately 12% over a mean time to malignant transformation of 4.3 years has recently been quoted. How reliable these data are, obtained from 14 non-related studies in a variety of different countries over a 40-year period, in determining a relevant risk calculation remains far from clear [1]. Mehenna et al. [1] had, in fact, actually identified a total of 2837 possible precancer progression papers in the literature over the 40-year search period in their attempt to establish a systematic review and undertake a meta-analysis to try and determine overall risk of cancer development. However, the fact that only 14 publications were ultimately deemed suitable for formal review in this way highlights the practical limitations of this type of research.

(A)

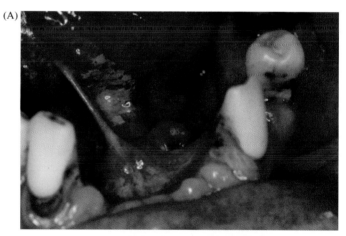

(B)

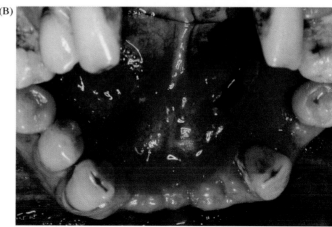

Figure 9.3 Widespread distribution of leukoplakic foci affecting the ventral tongue (A), and also involving the floor of the mouth and the lingual surface of mandibular alveolar mucosa (B). There is a high risk of malignant transformation in such a case, but it remains impossible to predict which site is most at risk.

It is important to note that Mehanna et al. emphasised that the only effective treatment for oral dysplastic lesions appears to be surgical excision. Although not eliminating the risk of cancer completely, excision does appear to decrease the risk of malignant transformation of potentially malignant lesions by more than a half [1]. These authors also observed a higher malignant transformation rate of 24.1% in severely dysplastic lesions compared with 10.3% for mild to moderately dysplastic ones. They were unable to comment on the relative risk in relation to other factors such as patient gender, smoking status, alcohol use and lesion site [1].

A number of observational, follow-up studies exist in the published literature. These are worth considering in some detail, not only to summarise our current knowledge base, but also to help appreciate the limitations of our real understanding of the risks of oral carcinogenesis in potentially malignant disorder cases.

Silverman et al. in a paper from 1984, reviewed 257 patients with oral leukoplakia who were followed for an average period of 7.2 years. They observed that, overall, 45 patients (or 17.5%) subsequently went on to develop a squamous cell carcinoma, usually within a 2-year observation period. However, only 22 of the 257 patients actually demonstrated dysplasia on initial microscopic examination so that the true transformation rate for dysplastic lesions was actually 36.4% [2]. These authors also noted that high risks for malignant transformation included non-smoking patients, females, lesions with red or erosive characteristics, verrucous hyperplastic lesions, and lesions exhibiting dysplasia on microscopy. In addition, they remarked that an increasing number of cancers were likely to be seen as the length of follow up increased [2].

Hogewind et al. in 1989 similarly observed an increased risk of oral cancer development in older, female patients by following 84 leukoplakia cases for an average period of 5 years. In total, three out of the 84 patients developed cancer, producing a malignant transformation rate of 3.6% [3].

Lumerman et al. in 1995 reported a 16% malignancy transformation rate: seven cases of cancer developed out of 44 patients with oral epithelial dysplasia, within a mean follow-up period of about 34 months. Two of the seven cancer patients in this series developed their tumours at sites distant from the original dysplasia [4]. Interestingly, these authors also combined the results of their study with four previous publications over the preceding 25 years and observed that whilst 6% of 65 patients who had their precancer lesions excised developed carcinoma, the figure rose to over 15% of 91 cases who received no treatment [4]. Clearly, there are significant limitations in combining unrelated studies, but it is interesting to note that Lumerman et al. clearly concluded that surgical intervention should be recommended for all patients presenting with oral dysplastic lesions.

In 1998 in a review of 166 patients with leukoplakia seen over a 24-year period, Schepman et al. observed that 20 patients (or 12% of cases) developed squamous cell carcinoma at a median time of 32 months of follow up, although no distinction was made in this study between same-site malignant transformation and carcinoma development elsewhere in the oral cavity [5]. Parameters associated with an increased risk of malignancy included female patients, non-smokers (especially females) and a non-homogeneous clinical appearance of individual lesions. The authors stated that patients who had 'any form of intervention' did not have a significantly lower risk of malignant transformation compared with non-intervention cases [5]. However, this was a highly retrospective study incorporating a variety of different treatment modalities instituted at varying times in the disease history rendering specific observations on the efficacy of treatments somewhat unreliable.

Cowan et al. in 2001 carried out a retrospective review of histopathology records over a 20-year period and estimated that 14% of 165 identifiable oral dysplastic lesions transformed to squamous cell carcinoma at an average interval from diagnosis of 48 months [6]. Whilst a number of interesting observations and suggestions were made by these authors, this study is clearly limited both by it being based upon histopathology laboratory data and also because of the highly retrospective nature of such data collection.

In reviewing 1458 Taiwanese patients who presented over a 10-year period with a variety of potentially malignant disorders, Hsue et al. reported an overall malignant transformation rate of 3% [7]. On closer inspection of the data, only 166 cases actually exhibited dysplasia and the majority of those showed only mildly dysplastic features; eight of these 166 cases progressed to malignancy, providing a transformation rate of nearer 4.8%. This again emphasises the limitations of such retrospective review studies even in the presence of apparently large numbers of patients.

In a more recent retrospective review of 207 patients presenting with oral epithelial dysplasia over a 16-year period, Arduino et al. in 2009 observed malignant transformation in 7.24% of cases (15 patients) occurring at a median time of about 30 months follow up. The vast majority of lesions studied showed mild dysplasia only, however, and the authors were unable to determine a predictive role for dysplasia severity [8]. A variety of uncoordinated treatment modalities were performed on 133 patients, including scalpel excisions and cryotherapy, whilst the remaining 74 patients underwent a 'wait and see' policy. Unfortunately, no clear rationale for any treatment decision appears to have been recorded and there seems to be a conspicuous lack of any cohesive or coordinated treatment protocol for precancer patients [8]. Perhaps unsurprisingly, in view of the above inconsistencies, the authors were unable to predict the risk of malignancy development, noting that neither the clinical type nor site of lesion, nor patient age, gender or risk factor behaviour influenced carcinogenesis, although non-homogeneous lesions were once again thought to be at an increased risk [8].

Ho et al. reviewed malignant transformation of potentially malignant disorders in a further Taiwanese population study of 148 male patients presenting over an 18-year period. There were, however, only 33 patients in this study with biopsy-proven epithelial dysplasia. Eight of these progressed to malignancy so that although the authors quoted an overall 7.6% transformation rate, the real percentage transformation for dyplastic lesions was actually 24% [9]. Whilst these authors noted that the tongue seems to be at particular risk of malignancy and that transformation is more common in the first 2–3 years after diagnosis [9], the heterogeneity of the study group, the lack of any treatment intervention and the small number of true dysplasia cases studied must question the overall relevance of this paper. However, Ho et al. do make an interesting point in their paper regarding the calculation of malignant transformation rates. Criticising the simple mathematical estimate of transformation using the number of malignant cases divided by the total number of study patients, they usefully emphasise that individual person—time malignant transformation rates are more appropriate calculations, particularly as the incidence of cancer is known to increase with the length of follow-up period [9].

Nonetheless, it is clearly important to stress that many published papers have quoted overall malignant transformation rates, varying from 3% to 17%, for heterogeneous patient populations often containing substantial numbers of lesions without dysplastic features. When these malignant transformation rates are recalculated using only dysplastic precursor lesions, the risk of malignancy increases to between 24% and 36%. Whilst it is recognised that lesions apparently without dysplasia may transform this is relatively rare, and most commentators have reported an increasing risk with the more severely dysplastic lesions, as summarised by Mehenna et al. [1].

The fundamental problem remains that all of the above studies are of highly variable quality, with different patient populations presenting with mixed dysplastic and non-dysplastic lesions, and inconsistent treatment and follow-up regimes. Similarly, and of considerable clinical significance, is that the actual site at which oral cancer develops is not clearly defined in many of the studies, thus failing to distinguish between site-specific malignant transformation and new-site cancer development.

Napier and Speight recently published an overview of the natural history of oral potentially malignant disorders. In relation to malignant transformation, they listed a number of possible factors predictive of cancer development [10]. These are summarised in Box 9.1 and include increased patient age, female patients, lesions present for a prolonged time, lesions arising in the floor of mouth, lateral tongue and retromolar regions, non-homogeneous leukoplakias and erythroplakias, dysplastic lesions in non-smokers, and large or multiple lesions [10].

Consensus opinion to date on oral precancer progression thus sadly offers very little in addition to that which we already know from our original and longstanding epidemiological observations that oral dysplastic lesions carry an increased risk of transformation to cancer. An annual malignant transformation rate of 1–2% has been suggested worldwide, although this calculation may actually be irrelevant when dealing with populations of patients presenting with truly dysplastic lesions where the risk of transformation appears considerably higher. Whilst it is probably true to state that carcinogenesis is more likely to occur in high-grade or severely dysplastic lesions, it is unfortunate that an accurate prediction of which patients or lesions will progress to malignancy is not yet possible in our clinical practices [10,11].

As a result, therefore, surgical excision of potentially malignant lesions is recommended to help decrease the risk of oral cancer development. It is relevant that most authors also stress the importance of regular clinic follow up and continued surveillance for all precancer patients [1].

Malignant transformation versus oral cancer development

As a result of detailed analyses of our Newcastle patient cohort studies, which were described in Chapter 8 and summarised in Table 8.1, we believe it is important to distinguish between two distinct types of invasive carcinoma presentation that may arise in potentially malignant disorder patients.

Firstly, there is *malignant transformation*, which is the change of a previously identified precancer lesion into an invasive squamous cell carcinoma at the same site as its precursor lesion.

Box 9.1 High-risk features for malignant transformation.

Patient factors
- Older patients

- Female gender

- Non-smoking patients with dysplastic lesions

Disease presentation
- Increased duration of clinical disorder

- Multiple lesion disease

Clinical appearance
- Erythroplakia

- Erythroleukoplakia

- Proliferative verrucous leukoplakia

- Non-homogeneous leukoplakia

- Erosive or ulcerated lesions

- Large, confluent lesions

Anatomical site
- Floor of mouth

- Ventrolateral tongue

- Retromolar region

- Gingiva

Histopathological features
- High-grade dysplasia

Secondly, there is *oral cancer development*, which is a term that should be used when patients with pre-existing or previously treated precancer lesions subsequently develop an invasive squamous cell carcinoma at new intra-oral sites, distant from their original presenting lesions.

A distinction between these two processes is fundamental because, as we have seen in Chapters 7 and 8, interventional treatment that excises individual oral precancer lesions may help to prevent malignant transformation at the site of the excised lesion. Several of our studies exhibit a 0% same-site transformation rate (see Table 8.1). This is an important longitudinal observation supporting surgical intervention because the majority of excised lesions in our studies exhibited either severe or moderate dysplasia on initial presentation, whilst the transformation rates for unexcised, truly dysplastic lesions in the studies described above varied between 24% and 36% [2,6,8,9]. However, oral cancer development at new oral sites still remains a risk for these patients, especially in the presence of ongoing risk factor behaviour, although it is encouraging that we have found this to be relatively low (approximately 2%) following interventional laser surgery (see Table 8.1).

The development of new-site carcinoma reflects, of course, the overall field change nature of oral potentially malignant disorders. The fact that patients are under active surveillance and regular clinic follow up post-laser treatment helps early recognition of such malignant change.

Whilst some authors cite any oral cancer development as a failure of interventional therapy, this is not only incorrect but oversimplifies the clinical situation. We firmly believe that prevention of malignant transformation (same-site cancer) can be achieved in the majority of patients by the excision of precursor lesions. As long as active surveillance and long-term follow up remain as mandatory components of interventional therapy, early signs of cancer development can also be recognised and further active surgical intervention facilitated.

Interventional laser surgery and oral cancer prevention

It is probably best, therefore, to consider any interventional management strategy as cyclical in nature, passing from active surgical excision through to a surveillance phase and returning back to surgical intervention upon diagnosis of additional precancer disease. It is thus a consistent and determined approach and applied rigorously to patients with potentially malignant disorders should ultimately lead to a reduced risk of invasive carcinoma development.

A considerable advantage of laser surgery is the ability to repeat excisions or ablations at the same site on a number of occasions. We have found that in the relatively small number of patients who develop persistent or recurrent precancer disease, multiple laser treatments – sometimes up to eight treatments at one site but separated by time for healing – are not only well tolerated by patients with minimal morbidity but ultimately can control and resolve recalcitrant disease.

Theoretical concerns have been raised that adjacent unstable or dysplastic mucosa may be excessively stimulated by laser treatments to a particular oral field, especially if repeated. However, this has not been our experience in any of the patient cohorts we have followed clinically.

A particularly difficult patient group to manage and follow up, of course, are those patients who present with multiple lesion disease. Although 'field mapping' improves diagnostic accuracy and rationalises treatment interventions, there is a significantly increased risk of oral cancer development in these patients as a result of more widespread field cancerisation. We followed 96 precancer patients who presented with 132 dysplastic oral lesions over a 5-year period. Seven patients were identified who developed an oral cancer, although in six of these cases the cancers arose at sites distinct from their excised lesions [12]. Whilst a malignant transformation rate of 3.8% (three out of 78 patients) was seen in single lesion disease, this rose to 22.2% (four out of 18 patients) for those presenting with multiple lesion disease [12].

Constant mucosal surveillance, perhaps utilising diagnostic adjunctive techniques, and early targeting of further disease with interventional laser, is again the most pragmatic and efficacious management strategy for such cases.

Newcastle 10-year follow-up study

Diajil (2011), in a detailed and comprehensive review of 100 single dysplastic lesion patients treated in Newcastle by laser surgery excision and followed up for 10 years (as described in Chapter 8), reported a malignant transformation rate of 5% for same-site cancer [13]. This is a higher transformation rate than we observed in our other cohort studies listed in Table 8.1, but probably reflects the increasing risk of disease progression and cancer development over a 10-year follow-up period. It does, however, provide us with a very important subgroup of patients to study in detail.

In general, oral cancers tended to occur at a mean time of 12 months after laser surgery and this is clearly shown in graph form in Figure 9.4. Most transformed disease tended to occur in middle-aged or older patients, with a higher proportion of females affected. Larger, non-homogeneous lesions, especially those arising on the floor of mouth, lateral tongue and retromolar regions, are particularly at risk. Current smokers and those consuming regular alcohol were at most risk of transformation [13]. These observations are highly consistent with the overall trends summarised and reported by Napier and Speight [10].

Oral cancer development, which we have defined as carcinoma arising at new intra-oral sites distant from precursor lesions, was seen in only two cases in Diajil's series. Both of these cases occurred nearly 5 years after successful laser excision of severely dysplastic lesions from ventrolateral tongue sites (Figure 9.5). Interestingly, both patients were non-smokers with only light alcohol consumption and both had shown multiple precancer lesion development at numerous intra-oral sites, which as we have already seen does seem to pose a higher risk for cancer development [12,13].

Diajil's observations again clearly emphasise the importance of long-term clinical follow up and active surveillance of inherently unstable oral mucosa in all oral potentially malignant disorder patients.

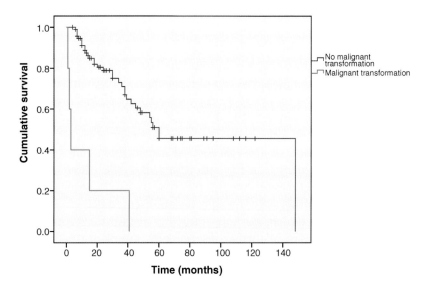

Figure 9.4 Kaplan–Meier survival analysis showing malignant same-site transformation, arising mainly within the first 12 months following laser surgery.

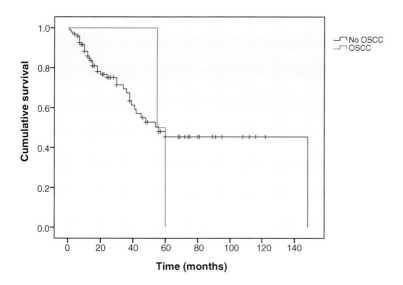

Figure 9.5 Kaplan–Meier survival analysis illustrating the development of oral squamous cell carcinoma (OSCC), or new-site disease, in two patients both occurring at around 5 years post-laser surgery.

High- and low-risk patients

In all types of precancer presentation the ability to distinguish individual patients at 'high risk' of cancer development from those at 'low risk' remains a fundamental goal. It would help concentrate diagnostic measures and rationalise therapeutic intervention at the earliest possible stages of clinical management.

Classically, of course, increased severity of dysplasia identified in potentially malignant lesion biopsies, increasing patient age at presentation, and heavy exposure to tobacco and alcohol are the most commonly quoted factors to be correlated with malignant transformation of precursor lesions [14]. As we have also seen, clinical lesion appearance in terms of non-homogeneous leukoplakias, erythroplakic lesions and erosive or ulcerated lesions are also thought to be high-risk features. These observations, however, are generalised and not always helpful in individual patient diagnosis and management strategies. Further work is necessary to try to distinguish reliable risk stratification systems, ideally by combining both histopathological features and clinical data.

Work is ongoing in these important areas and this is a vitally important area for future research into oral potentially malignant disease. We will therefore return to this important topic in more detail in the next chapter of this book.

Clinical signs of oral squamous cell carcinoma

In the absence of tailored individual patient management strategies, we have already demonstrated how important active surveillance is in the long-term management of potentially malignant disorder patients. It is vitally important during patient follow up to try to recognise clinical signs and elicit symptoms suggestive of carcinoma development at the earliest possible stage. A high index of suspicion is essential to alert clinicians to recognise malignant transformation.

Box 9.2 summarises the salient, but often quite varied, clinical features seen in oral squamous cell carcinoma presentation, although it remains a significant

Box 9.2 Mnemonic for the clinical signs of oral squamous cell carcinoma.

- Oral ulceration (non-healing)
- Raised, everted, exophytic, indurated lesions
- Abnormal swellings
- Loss of tongue mobility, dysarthria, otalgia
- Cauliflower-like or warty growths
- Abnormal, localised tooth mobility
- Non-healing tooth sockets
- Colour changes in mucosa – red, white or speckled patches
- Erosive, raw mucosal patches
- Reduced or altered oro-facial sensation

problem that patients often remain unaware of such changes until lesions have reached an advanced stage. Figure 9.6 illustrates a typical clinical scenario with an established squamous cell carcinoma presenting in the anterior floor of mouth and mandibular alveolus. Late-presenting squamous cell carcinoma, of course, risks local and destructive invasion of oral and facial tissues together with cervical lymph node metastases and a resultant increase in both patient morbidity and mortality.

Overall 5-year survival rates for intra-oral cancers remain at around 50% and, even with real advances in ablative treatments, reconstructive surgery and chemoradiotherapy techniques, have not significantly improved in recent years. Oral squamous cell carcinoma is thus a lethal disease with local tumour recurrence, metachronous primary tumour development, and distant metastases all contributing to treatment failure.

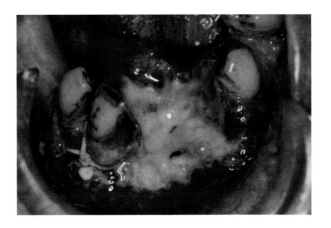

Figure 9.6 Infiltrative, irregular, indurated and ulcerative squamous cell carcinoma presenting in the floor of the mouth and mandibular alveolus. There is adjacent leukoplakia overlying the submandibular ducts which predated the invasive carcinoma development.

Diagnosis and management of 'unexpected malignancy'

It is obvious from the above comments that the identification and elimination of oral squamous cell carcinoma at the earliest possible stage must be a priority for oral oncologists. We have previously emphasised the efficacy of interventional laser surgery as both a diagnostic and treatment modality in oral precancer management [15], so it is logical to consider its role in early cancer recognition.

We carried out a retrospective review of 169 patients who presented over a 5-year period with single, new, oral dysplastic lesions excised by laser. We found that in 15 cases (or approximately 9%) an 'unexpected' invasive squamous cell carcinoma was discovered upon histopathological examination of the excision biopsy specimens [16]. Interestingly, whilst no distinct demographic or clinicopathological features could reliably identify patients at risk of 'unexpected' carcinoma, the majority were found in lesions with a previous incisional biopsy diagnosis of either severe or moderate dysplasia.

Laser interventions to excise lesions were all carried out within 6–8 weeks following incisional biopsy. It is probable that these foci of carcinoma were present and missed at initial biopsy, possibly because of sampling errors. In all cases the 'unexpected' carcinomas were completely excised by laser with margins greater then 5 mm. Whilst mean laser excision specimens measured 26.7 mm long by 15.2 mm wide by 5.8 mm deep, the foci of carcinomas were quite small with mean dimensions of only 2.9 mm diameter by 1.8 mm deep. It is especially pertinent to emphasise that none of these patients developed local tumour recurrence or regional metastasis during a mean 36-month follow-up period [16].

Interventional laser surgery and the complete excision of potentially malignant lesions, therefore, not only helps establish a definitive diagnosis and facilitate treatment of dysplastic lesions but is also efficacious in the management of early neoplastic lesions, especially at a stage when malignant change is clinically undetectable.

It remains unknown, of course, whether all oral squamous cell carcinomas are preceded by identifiable potentially malignant changes. Through the years some authors have suggested that the varying clinical outcomes observed in cancer patients may be due to different carcinogenic pathways. For example, more aggressive carcinomas may arise de novo from clinically normal mucosa, whilst those developing from precancer potentially malignant lesions might exhibit a slower and less aggressive course [6]. This is highly speculative, though, and there is no real convincing evidence in the literature for such a hypothesis.

Certainly, however, our finding of 'unexpected' carcinomas in 9% of excised dysplastic lesions does seem to support the progression model for oral carcinogenesis, as outlined in Chapter 3. Other workers have also observed that 5–10% of oral leukoplakias may contain frankly invasive, but clinically unrecognised, carcinoma upon excision biopsy. This similarly supports the concept of initially dysplastic tissue ultimately transforming to a neoplastic state [17]. Such observations lend increasing weight to our hypothesis that clinically recognisable precursor lesions offer a window of therapeutic opportunity to intervene to prevent and in some cases actually treat early oral squamous carcinoma. Our experience of treating and following up such patients tells us that the early excision of an 'unexpected' carcinoma is indeed an effective treatment, with minimal morbidity, a disease-free follow-up period and no obvious compromised clinical outcome following, effectively, an 'unplanned' cancer excision.

All patients with an 'unexpected' carcinoma diagnosis are subsequently seen in our multidisciplinary head and neck clinics to review their pathological diagnoses and reassess excision specimen details. They are then imaged, as appropriate, and retrospectively staged in terms of their oral cancer disease as accurately as is possible for post-surgical excision cases. Further treatment interventions and follow-up strategies are agreed by the full multidisciplinary team, as for all head and neck oncology patients.

Prognosis for the 'transformed' patient

What, then, is the overall significance for the patient whose precancer lesion transforms into a malignancy, especially in terms of their long-term clinical outcome? Unfortunately, there are no accurate data sets available to comment definitively on this issue. Indeed, the late clinical presentation of many oral cancers in patients who are usually irregular dental attenders makes it difficult to ascertain the true number of tumours that may arise from potentially detectable precursor lesions.

Anecdotally, in our dysplasia clinics in Newcastle, we have found that patients with oral precancer who do transform can do very well so long as they are prepared to address their individual risk factor behaviours and attend for regular and careful specialist follow up. Both recurrent and further precancer development, as well as metachronous primary squamous cell carcinomas, may develop in these patients but a structured and active clinical surveillance programme to precisely identify mucosal abnormalities helps facilitate early diagnosis and highlight further sites that may be undergoing carcinogenesis.

In a number of individual cases, often elderly, female patients with multifocal disease, we have found that determined and repeated laser treatments to areas of persistent, recurrent or further mucosal disease can ultimately bring about complete clinical resolution. This may require multiple treatment episodes over time but can be applied to both precancer lesions and early invasive malignancies although, particularly for the latter, this must be very carefully monitored.

It remains, of course, virtually impossible to offer reliable long-term prognoses to any individual oral cancer patient. However, we believe that a management protocol that emphasises regular and accurate clinical follow up, allows oral mucosal surveillance and early recognition, and immediate excision of malignant or potentially malignant lesions will undoubtedly reduce morbidity and should help improve long-term prognosis.

Summary

Oral potentially malignant disorders retain a variable and unpredictable risk of squamous cell carcinoma development. Such malignant disease can arise at the site of precancer lesion presentation as a malignant transformation, or as new disease at distinct oral sites as a result of field cancerisation. No reliable clinicopathological features accurately predict the risk of such carcinogenesis. Interventional surgery to excise precancer lesions, however, appears to reduce the incidence of same-site transformation, but new-site cancer development still remains a risk. In addition, surgical excision of precancer lesions offers an opportunity to diagnose and effectively treat occult invasive carcinomas at a stage when otherwise clinically unidentifiable. Irrespective of treatment intervention, long-term patient follow up and active surveillance is important for all cases as there appears to be an increasing risk of cancer development over time.

References

1. Mehanna HM, Rattay T, Smith J, McConkey CC. Treatment and follow-up of oral dysplasia – a systematic review and meta-analysis. *Head Neck* 2009; 31: 1600–1609.
2. Silverman S, Gorsky M, Lozada F. Oral leukoplakia and malignant transformation. A follow-up study of 257 patients. *Cancer* 1984; 53: 563–568.
3. Hogewind WFC, van der Kwast WAM, van der Waal I. Oral leukoplakia, with emphasis on malignant transformation: a follow-up study of 46 patients. *J Craniomaxillofac Surg* 1989; 17: 128–133.
4. Lumerman H, Freedman P, Kerpel S. Oral epithelial dysplasia and the development of invasive squamous cell carcinoma. *Oral Surg Oral Med Oral Pathol* 1995; 79: 321–329.
5. Schepman KP, van der Meij EH, Smeele LE, van der Waal I. Malignant transformation of oral leukoplakia: a follow-up study of a hospital-based population of 166 patients with oral leukoplakia from the Netherlands. *Oral Oncol* 1998; 34: 270–275.
6. Cowan GC, Gregg TA, Napier SS, McKenna SM, Kee F. Potentially malignant oral lesions in Northern Ireland: a 20-year population-based perspective of malignant transformation. *Oral Dis* 2001; 7: 18–24.
7. Hsue S-S, Wang W-C, Chen C-H, Lin C-C, Chen Y-K, Lin L-M. Malignant transformation in 1458 patients with potentially malignant oral mucosal disorders: a follow-up study based in a Taiwanese hospital. *J Oral Pathol Med* 2007; 36: 25–29.
8. Arduino PG, Surace A, Carbone M, Elia A, Massolini G, Gandolfo S, Broccoletti R. Outcome of oral dysplasia: a retrospective hospital-based study of 207 patients with a long follow-up. *J Oral Pathol Med* 2009; 38: 540–544.
9. Ho PS, Chen PL, Warnakulasuriya S, Shieh TY, Chen YK, Huang IY. Malignant transformation of oral potentially malignant disorders in males: a retrospective study. *Cancer* 2009; 9: 260.
10. Napier SS, Speight PM. Natural history of potentially malignant oral lesions and conditions: an overview of the literature. *J Oral Pathol Med* 2000; 37: 1–10.
11. van der Waal I. Potentially malignant disorders of the oral and oropharyngeal mucosa: present concepts of management. *Oral Oncol* 2010; 46: 423–425.
12. Hamadah O, Goodson ML, Thomson PJ. Clinicopathological behaviour of multiple oral dysplastic lesions compared with that of single lesions. *Br J Oral Maxillofac Surg* 2010; 48: 503–506.
13. Diajil A. Personal communication, 2011.
14. Bosatra A, Bussani R, Silvestri F. From epithelial dysplasia to squamous carcinoma in the head and neck region: an epidemiological assessment. *Acta Otolaryngol (Stockh)* 1997; Suppl 527: 47–48.
15. Thomson PJ, Wylie J. Interventional laser surgery: an effective surgical and diagnostic tool in oral precancer management. *Int J Oral Maxillofac Surg* 2002; 31: 145–153.
16. Goodson ML, Thomson PJ. Management of oral carcinoma: benefits of early precancerous intervention. *Br J Oral Maxillofac Surg* 2011; 49: 88–91.
17. Holmstrup P, Vedtofte P, Reibel J, Stoltze K. Oral premalignant lesions: is a biopsy reliable? *J Oral Pathol Med* 2007; 36: 262–266.

10 The Future

Peter Thomson and Michaela L. Goodson

Introduction

Thus far in this book we have tried to concisely review our current understanding of the presentation, diagnosis, management and clinical outcomes for oral potentially malignant disorders. In doing so, it will no longer surprise the reader that it is very clear that there remain many unanswered questions and fundamental problems with our present knowledge base. A list of these limitations and the salient difficulties in our approach to oral precancer diagnosis and management is summarised in Box 10.1, together with a number of potential solutions that may help to address these problems.

In this chapter, therefore, we will attempt to look towards the future to see just how some of these important issues may be resolved. It is highly likely, though, that attempts to establish the true carcinogenic risk for oral potentially malignant lesions will be the subject of epidemiological, diagnostic, pathological, molecular and translational research for many years to come. The precise interplay of these factors is a complex process, and malignant transformation is most probably the result of a combination of intrinsic and extrinsic influences acting both synchronously and metachronously in any individual patient. Undoubtedly, however, it will only be by gaining a better understanding of the mechanisms involved in oral carcinogenesis that we will be able to improve prevention, early diagnosis, treatment and prognosis for both oral precancer and ultimately invasive squamous cell carcinoma itself.

Central to future developments in oral oncology will be the need to advance our knowledge of molecular biology. As our ability to identify molecular alterations associated with various disease states increases, the need to analyse these for diagnostic and therapeutic purposes grows. The human genome, which was first draft sequenced in 2001, contains over 30 000 genes packed into 23 pairs of chromosomes, with around 40 of them involved in the control of cell replication and proliferation. As we discussed in Chapter 3, loss of cell cycle control and abnormal proliferative activity is in many ways a fundamental hallmark of oral carcinogenesis and a more detailed study of these cell cycle

---

Box 10.1 Current problems and potential solutions in oral potentially malignant disorder management.

Current problems
- Non-specific precancer diagnosis with no reliable prediction of clinical behaviour

- No ability to determine future disease progression

- Unpredictable risk of oral malignancy

- Difficulty in determining the efficacy of treatment interventions

Solutions
- Individual patient profiling at the biomolecular level

- Targeted and effective interventional treatment with minimal morbidity

- Reduced risk of malignant transformation and cancer development

---

progression genes may help in future studies of tumour growth rates and the prediction of aggressive clinical behaviour.

Whilst numerous techniques are now available to study the molecular biology of carcinogenesis at both the genetic (genomic) or protein expression (proteomic) level, it is salutary to note that very few scientific advances have, to date, found routine application in the clinical setting. The ultimate aim of genotype-based predictive tests must be, of course, the ability to stratify risk, determine prognosis and thus personalise therapeutic intervention at an individual patient level [1].

In this chapter we will widen our discussion and look at ways in which both scientific advancement and more generalised approaches to health care may aid in the future prevention, diagnosis and treatment of oral potentially malignant disorders. We will also consider some possible future research directions that may help improve our understanding of oral precancer disease.

Prevention of oral precancer

Whilst there are still no universally agreed management strategies for treating established potentially malignant lesions, we have presented in this book an interventional management technique based upon excision laser surgery. To date this appears one of the best studied and most efficacious diagnostic and treatment options for oral precancer.

Primary prevention, however, must be considered as the initial and perhaps most important strategy in trying to stop the development of a potentially malignant disorder in the first place, rather than surgical attempts to eliminate the disease once it has become clinically apparent. As seen and emphasised in preceding chapters, we also believe that surgical intervention remains important and retains clear practical benefits in terms of both secondary and tertiary preventive strategies.

In the future, with the rates of new oral cancer cases rising, it will become increasingly important to strengthen our efforts to facilitate primary prevention of oral potentially malignant disease.

Tobacco and alcohol use

Tobacco has been shown both in the developing and developed world to be the commonest risk factor for oral cancer and potentially malignant lesions. However, most smokers do not actually develop oral cancer, which not only confounds the advice we give our patients but also, of course, underlines the importance of other, presumably inherent susceptibilities or pre-existing genetic factors.

There is definite evidence that once lesions have arisen, cessation of smoking may result in the clinical resolution of oral potentially malignant lesions. Importantly, this may also help prevent further disease arising after treatment. Thus, greater and improved emphasis on smoking cessation techniques and nicotine replacement therapy remains highly pertinent in modern clinical practice. This is probably most effective if provided directly to patients as part of specialist advice in dedicated dysplasia clinics (see Chapter 7).

It is our belief that centralisation of oral potentially malignant disorder patients in a dedicated clinic provides the optimum management strategy. Within such clinics, consistent, continually reinforced, specialist advice and treatment can be available together with multidisciplinary support, particularly for identifying and modifying risk factor behaviour. In the future it would be sensible for dedicated oral precancer clinics to be established to concentrate clinical experience, facilitate rigorous audit, develop research protocols and encourage new treatment trials. This would replace the present arrangement whereby patients attend a variety of different surgical or medical clinics dependent primarily upon local preferences or upon historical clinic arrangements.

Unfortunately, despite increased awareness of smoking as a risk factor and some significant reductions in smoking behaviour, we must recognise that there is a worldwide rise in the incidence of oral cancer. Alarmingly, this seems particularly to be the case for younger patients aged less than 50 years. It is possible that the substantial increases in alcohol consumption reported to be occurring in most developed countries may be partly responsible for this. Separating the carcinogenic effects of tobacco from alcohol remains difficult as most smokers also consume alcohol, so the precise effects of alcohol and tobacco either alone or synergistically are difficult to determine. There is no doubt, however, that opportunities for clinicians to offer advice to patients on reducing alcohol consumption should be taken and may well prove effective in longer term preventive strategies.

There is increasing awareness that all clinicians should become competent in recognising harmful alcohol drinking in their patients and be able to appropriately offer intervention, in much the same way as smoking cessation therapy. For alcohol, these may include cognitive behavioural therapies, effective and assisted alcohol withdrawal protocols and the promotion of abstinence [2]. Similarly, the recognition that harmful alcohol drinking and dependence is perhaps more akin to a drug addition rather than a socially acceptable habit may ultimately help in informing populations. There is no doubt that public awareness campaigns to prevent drink driving, targeting young drinkers to prevent chronic alcohol abuse and government policies to raise the minimum price for alcoholic beverages have been beneficial and have influenced public behaviour in a positive manner in recent years.

Human papillomavirus

Recent studies have suggested that the human papillomavirus (HPV), especially type 16, may play a causal role in a subgroup of primarily oropharyngeal, especially tonsillar and base of tongue, squamous cell carcinomas. There has been a dramatic rise in this type of oropharyngeal cancer over recent years with HPV positive cancers occurring in young, non smoking and non drinking patients. This may be a new and distinct disease entity, possibly related to high-risk sexual behaviour such as increased numbers of partners and oral–genital sex. Despite the presence of often large cervical nodal metastases, however, HPV-positive cases tend to respond better to chemoradiotherapy treatments than HPV-negative patients, although smoking appears to significantly worsen their clinical outcome [3].

The role of HPV in intra-oral cancer and oral potentially malignant lesions, especially for floor of mouth and ventrolateral tongue lesions, is poorly defined at the present time and will require further research. It may be that HPV plays a role during the early stages of oral carcinogenesis or may simply be a 'passenger' in morphologically altered tissues. However, it is very likely that well informed patients will want to know their HPV status in the future and this may have a direct effect on clinical management decisions. Meanwhile, the role of the recently introduced female-only HPV vaccination programme in influencing oral cancer disease presentation remains to be seen [3].

Dietary factors and healthy lifestyle choices

Epidemiological evidence surrounding the role of diet with regard to the development of oral potentially malignant lesions and oral cancer remains difficult to assess. The literature suggests a causative or contributory role for low fruit and vegetable intake in oral carcinogenesis. Diets vary tremendously around the world, of course, and the many confounding effects – such as high levels of tobacco smoking and the malnutrition consequent upon excessive alcohol consumption – complicate accurate dietary assessments in patient care.

However, it is likely that future preventive strategies will emphasise healthy, well balanced diets for many types of cancer prevention as well as general health promotion advice on losing weight, regular exercise and responsible sexual health. In the future, all health care professionals will be expected to increasingly engage patients in active discussions on personal habits and risk factor behaviour before moving firmly towards encouraging active patient participation in health living schemes [4].

Increasingly, public health promotion schemes such as 'Mouth Cancer Awareness Week' and 'Mouth Cancer Action Month' in the UK have tried to raise the profile of oral cancer to the general public, whilst also developing a greater public understanding of the links between oral and general health. Whether such campaigns will have an effect on clinical disease presentation in the long term is difficult to say as unfortunately, like many public health screening programmes, the people at most risk of disease rarely access such programmes and almost never present for health advice or preventive oral examination.

Nonetheless, it is likely that these public awareness campaigns will continue and they are, of course, to be encouraged. Current advice to prevent oral cancer and information provided to patients to accompany such programmes are summarised in Box 10.2. There is now a clear emphasis on a healthy diet, exercise and sexual health alongside more traditional advice on tobacco and alcohol use.

Early diagnosis of potentially malignant disease

We have already discussed the significant limitations inherent in trying to screen the general population for oral disease and the difficulties in identifying and

---

Box 10.2 Advice to prevent oral cancer.

- Stop smoking and avoid all forms of tobacco use

- Reduce or avoid alcohol intake, and ensure alcohol-free days every so often

- Eat healthily, with plenty of fresh fruit and vegetables in daily diet

- Maintain a healthy weight and avoid obesity

- Exercise moderately on most days of the week

- Maintain sexual health and practice safe sex using condoms and barriers

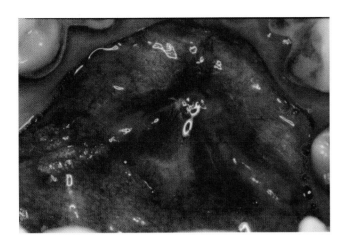

Figure 10.1 Floor of mouth mucosa demonstrating a small patch of homogeneous leukoplakia anteriorly over the opening of the submandibular duct, together with an irregular, warty, non-homogeneous lesion sited more posteriorly.

targeting high-risk groups for diagnostic intervention. It is assumed, and not unreasonably, that early diagnosis of oral potentially malignant disorders is desirable. This is based upon the hypothesis that once diagnosed, prompt intervention will stop the disease process and prevent oral cancer development. We have already seen that controversy exists as to whether either of the aforementioned aims can realistically be achieved for every patient. However, when the consequences of squamous cell carcinoma development in the oral cavity are so potentially disastrous, both in terms of patient morbidity and mortality, efforts to improve the prompt identification of precancer and early invasive oral carcinoma must be encouraged.

Clinical examination of the oral cavity remains first and foremost amongst the diagnostic techniques undertaken to identify suspicious oral lesions. Figure 10.1 illustrates the sometimes quite subtle mucosal changes, as seen in the floor of the mouth, which may be the first indications of precancer disease. To improve accuracy in distinguishing individuals who do or do not have malignant or potentially malignant disease, however, requires further investigation such as the use of biopsy for histopathological and/or cytological examination.

It is unlikely that any of the newer diagnostic aids reviewed in Chapter 5 will supplant standard clinical examination and incisional biopsy – which remain fundamental to the diagnosis of any suspicious oral lesion. These newer techniques are, however, proving to be useful adjuncts in specialist dysplasia clinics (see Chapters 4 and 7). Multicentre, randomised controlled clinical trials are needed to further investigate the precise role of, for example, light-based detection systems, exfoliative cytology and molecular biomarker testing.

Interventional management strategies in the future

We have outlined in the preceding chapters the efficacy of interventional laser surgery in the diagnosis and management of oral precancer and early invasive cancer, as illustrated in Figure 10.2. Unfortunately the natural history of potentially malignant disorders is both long and variable and lesions that have apparently disappeared following treatment, if followed up long enough, may recur. Perhaps of even greater biological significance is the realisation that the development of further or new-site disease may be observed. The structure of an interventional management protocol provides an important active surveillance phase post treatment that is especially important and relevant in addressing the long-term consequences of oral potentially malignant disease.

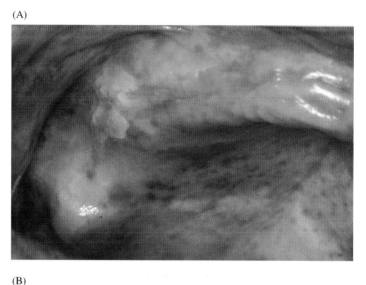

Figure 10.2 Laser excision of a leukoplakic lesion arising at the labial commisure.

Unfortunately, we have also found a subgroup of patients who present with widespread multifocal precancer disease, sometimes involving very large areas of oral mucosa, who are at even higher risk of cancer development. A typical clinical example of multiple lesion disease is illustrated in Figure 10.3. These cases require a very different management strategy to those with solitary

(A)

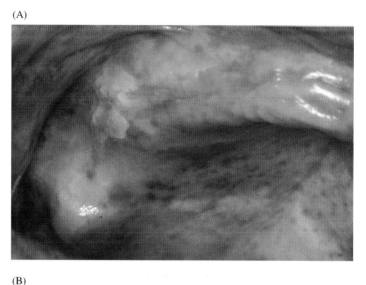

(B)

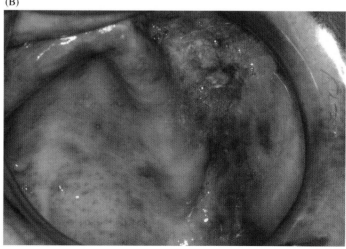

Figure 10.3 Edentulous patient presenting with multiple lesion disease showing non-homogeneous leukoplakia on the maxillary alveolus (A) and eryrthroleukoplakia involving the buccal sulcus on the contralateral side (B).

Type of therapy	Mechanism of action
Gene therapy	
Addition	Introduction of tumour suppressor genes such as p27, p53 and retinoblastoma gene
Deletion	Removal of defective oncogenes
Suicide	Cytotoxin production in target cells
Antisense RNA	Prevention of oncogene activity
Viral vectors	
Retrovirus	Oncolytic viruses only replicate in and destroy tumour cells
Adenoviruses	
Adeno-associated viruses	
Herpesviruses	
Immunotherapy	
Interleukins	Increased immune response to tumour
T lymphocytes	
Natural killer cells	
Angiogenesis inhibition	
VEGF inhibitor	Inhibition of angiogenesis, tumour growth and metastasis

VEGF, vascular endothelial growth factor.

Table 10.1 Future management strategies.

lesions, sometimes involving field mapping biopsies, targeted laser surgery and often repeated treatment interventions.

It also remains frustratingly difficult for clinicians that, despite a plethora of new potential biomarkers of disease behaviour being identified in recent years, we remain unable to predict clinical outcomes for any individual patient or precancer lesion that we treat.

Future interventional management strategies demand a greater understanding of the development and natural history of precancer and ideally will involve not just localised oral treatments but also a more systemic and longer lasting approach to patient management. It is interesting, therefore, to review current research into novel therapies for oral cancer and precancer, and Table 10.1 summarises a number of potential therapeutic interventions that may be of use in the management of potentially malignant oral disorders in the future.

Of particular interest for future treatments are the *gene therapy* techniques in which target cells in a patient are genetically modified, either by introducing new or by modifying existing genetic material. The particular aim of these approaches is to help fight disease without producing toxic effects on surrounding normal tissue [5]. In essence, gene therapy may involve the stimulation of tumour suppressor genes in addition therapy to deactivate carcinogenesis, or genes can be introduced into cells to generate toxic products as suicide therapies. In deletion or excision therapy the aim is to formally remove dysfunctional oncogenes from the target cells [5].

Viral vectors have also been proposed as oncolytic anti-cancer agents, and by observed mechanisms whereby viruses will replicate only in tumour cells may prove to be the most practical method of gene therapy. ONYX-015, for example, is a replication competent adenovirus that selectively replicates in and causes lysis of cells with deficient p53 activity. p53 is significantly affected in squamous epithelial cells during oral carcinogenesis and there is increasing evidence that reintroduction of functional p53 into tumours may well be of therapeutic benefit [6]. Interestingly, in 2003 Rudin et al. reported a small clinical trial in which 22 patients with premalignant oral lesions used a mouthwash containing ONYX-015 as a treatment modality [7]. Unfortunately, the results were somewhat disappointing with only two patients free of clinical lesions 2 years following therapy. Although such local treatment was well tolerated with minimal side effects, the therapeutic actions were only transient with a limited p53 response [7].

So, despite using modern technology, the use of a genetically engineered mouthwash appears to offer little improvement from the failed medical interventions that we have already reviewed in Chapter 7. It also similarly fails to address the inherently provisional nature of incisional biopsy diagnosis and the risk of treating unrecognised early squamous carcinoma all of which, as we have previously seen, can be efficiently managed by formal laser excision of precancer lesions.

Other workers have reported the use of an attenuated herpes simplex virus, OncoVEX, to preferentially infect and lyse head and neck cancer cells, subsequently releasing proteins to help stimulate the immune system [8]. Clinical trials are underway in combination with chemoradiotherapy treatments, but it remains to be seen how effective this therapy will actually prove to be and indeed whether it has a specific role in precancer treatment.

Immunotherapy is a novel approach being trialled primarily in advanced cancer disease and is based upon the observed ability of host defences to damage and destroy malignancies. Some oral cancer patients have been shown to exhibit depressed immune cell function, so that the aim of immunotherapy is to increase the patient's immune response to the tumour. Unfortunately, a tumour-specific vaccine for head and neck carcinoma has so far proved somewhat elusive, and whether such an approach will have a useful role in marshalling a local response to dysplastic epithelium remains to be seen [9].

Individualised patient treatments: biomarkers and targeted chemoprevention

We have tried in our clinics to delineate patients thought to be at 'high risk' or 'low risk' from their oral potentially malignant disorders. Based upon a combination of their age, gender, medical background and risk factors, together with the site, size, clinical appearance and histopathology of their presenting oral lesions, this is designed to identify those cases requiring urgent interventional treatment to try to prevent cancer development. We believe that this is an appropriate and pragmatic approach to current patient management, but it remains a somewhat crude decision-making tool. In the future, treatments should ideally become much more individualised and patient specific based upon molecular profiling and targeted therapeutic intervention.

Molecular targeted therapy aims specifically to inhibit tumour growth and metastasis by targeting the tumour microenvironment or vasculature, or focusing on specific protein or signal transduction pathways in neoplastic or dysplastic tissue, leaving normal cells unaffected. In recent years a variety of molecular targeted chemoprevention techniques have been developed. Unfortunately evidence to support any of these is very limited, few have been subjected to randomised controlled trials and little work has been carried out in oral potentially malignant disease.

A number of clinical trials have been based upon the inhibition of the epidermal growth factor receptor (EGFR), which is known to be overexpressed in oral squamous cell carcinoma. Cetuximab, for example, is a monoclonal antibody against EGFR and has been used, often in combination with chemoradiotherapy, in effectively treating head and neck carcinomas.

Angiogenesis, by definition, is the formation of new vessels from existing vasculature and undoubtedly plays a critical role in tumour development. It is known to be stimulated by growth factors released from neoplastic tissue, such as the vascular endothelial growth factor (VEGF) family, that facilitate the growth of new vessels into developing tumour tissue [10]. Bevacizumab is a monoclonal antibody that binds to VEGF, blocking its interaction with VEGF receptors. There are suggestions that such angiogenesis inhibition may have a therapeutic role in head and neck cancer [11]. Whether inhibition of angiogenesis reduces the risk of severely dysplastic tissue transforming into invasive carcinoma, however, remains speculative but it is certainly an area of potential research interest for the future.

Epidemiological studies have suggested that the regular use of non-steroidal anti-inflammatory drugs (NSAIDs) may have a protective effect against cancer development. Cyclo-oxygenase 2 (COX-2) is the probable target of NSAIDs and is an enzyme known to be upregulated in tumours. Its actions, probably mediated via prostaglandin production, have been shown to increase cell proliferation, invasion and angiogenesis whilst at the same time decreasing apopotosis and host immune responses [10]. Unfortunately, COX-2-specific NSAID use risks a number of unwanted cardiovascular thrombotic side effects and clinical trials, which have not to date shown especially promising results for oral precancer management, have slowed while safer alternatives are sought. Incidentally, we previously investigated the influence of NSAID use in 30 oral precancer patients, but found no significant difference in dysplasia grading, p53 activity or clinical outcome following laser excision of oral lesions when we compared aspirin users with non-aspirin users [12].

Preliminary work on targeted genetics, interleukin-mediated therapy, monoclonal antibodies directed at carcinoembryonic antigen, and peroxisome proliferator-activated receptor inhibitors (PPARIs) has also been carried out in various studies. These suggest that there may be a number of other potential roles to further investigate in precancer chemoprevention.

In summary, we believe that a number of possible biomarker chemopreventive targets may exist. However, whilst a number of clinical trials are currently underway assessing the possible benefits of these drugs, it is likely to be some time before any can be put into routine use as chemopreventive agents for the management of oral carcinogenesis. In the future, we look forward to being able to offer patients a range of evidence-based individualised management options tailored to specific risk factors, histopathological classifications and biomarker status. For the time being, however, oral precancer treatment is likely to continue in its current mode with management strategies being guided by clinician preference, experience and the pragmatism of excising potentially malignant tissue.

Future research directions

Scientific research

The main thrusts of scientific research into oral carcinogenesis will probably be dependent upon further advances into the understanding of molecular biological changes during oral carcinogenesis. Changes within DNA (genome), RNA

Box 10.3 Newly emerging diagnostic molecular technology.

DNA (genome)
- DNA sequencing
- Array comparative genomic hybridisation (aCGH)
- Single nucleotide polymorphisms (SNPs)

Gene expression (mRNA/transcriptome)
- Microarrays based on cDNA/oligonucleotides
- Serial analysis of gene expression (SAGE)

Proteins (proteome)
- Immunohistochemistry
- Two-dimensional polyacrylamide gel electrophoresis (2D PAGE)
- Mass spectrometry
- Protein microarray platforms

(transcription) and protein (proteome) levels within precancerous tissue should become increasingly identifiable and those predisposing to malignant transformation may then be utilised as predictive biomarkers. Box 10.3 summarises the range of emerging diagnostic molecular technologies that in the future will allow high throughput screening for thousands of disease-related biomolecules in test samples [13].

Genomic research It is recognised that predisposition to disease is influenced by genetic make up so a key priority in scientific research must be to try to understand the clinical relevance of both the form and function of individual genes, not only in healthy but especially in diseased tissue.

Microarray technology is a newer method of high throughput screening of gene expression. Automated and miniaturised analysis of multiple, tiny cores of tissue on small glass slides using labelled DNA probes allows literally tens of thousands of specific RNA or DNA sequences to be detected simultaneously. Characteristic patterns of gene expression are recognised. These may have practical applications as diagnostic, therapeutic or prognostic tools, particularly when tissue is available from large clinical trials in which treatments and clinical outcome are well documented [14]. It is highly likely that in the future microarray work will be increasingly applied to the analysis of dysplastic and neoplastic tissue.

A range of other genome-based abnormalities have been identified and suggested as possible markers of carcinogenesis particularly in relation to cell division. These include mitochondrial DNA mutations and shortening of telomeres, which may lead to replicative cell senescence, chromosomal instability and increased cancer risk [15,16].

Proteomic research This type of research work is designed to characterise the presence and activity of translated gene products in normal and diseased conditions. This is a promising area of future research because it is, after all, primarily abnormal protein function in cells that produces disease.

Traditionally, as we have seen in preceding chapters, *immunohistochemical* techniques have been used in identifying in situ localisation of protein products in pathological tissue sections. Increasingly, however, with the introduction of *mass spectrometry*, thousands of distinct proteins and their functional networks can be identified and applied to a variety of tissue, blood and body fluid analyses [17]. Human body fluid proteome (HBFP) analysis, for example, has recently been proposed as an important tool in the search for clinically relevant disease biomarkers. Whilst the identification of both full-length and partially degraded forms of mRNA in saliva has suggested that a saliva-based test for oral cancer detection may be possible in the future.

All such techniques, however, will still be heavily reliant upon longitudinal cohort studies of individual patients presenting with oral potentially malignant disorders and will require detailed and comprehensive long-term clinical outcome data.

Morphonomics   We have already commented how useful it is to preserve intact the structural hierarchy of oral mucosal tissue to aid in the interpretation of the biomolecular changes observed in dysplastic tissue. Morphonomic research is thus designed to relate genomic and proteomic data to the morphological changes in histopathology specimens. Modern *laser capture microdissection* techniques use low-energy, infrared laser pulses to dissect unfixed tissue. This allows defined tissue samples, or even individual cells, to be harvested from thin histological sections, thus facilitating a structural based analysis of homogeneous cell populations. Application of these techniques may well be particularly relevant to the future analysis of dysplastic tissue and its progression to an invasive malignancy.

Bioinformatics   The use of computer technology and mathematical analyses to handle the ever increasing amounts of biomedical data is a central requirement for successful future research in cancer and precancer. Microarray platforms and proteomic analyses, as exampled above, literally provide data on tens of thousands of genes and proteins from multiple tissue samples and can only be pragmatically analysed by computerised methodologies. Bioinformatics expertise will thus be an essential prerequisite in the future, to harness these enormous data sets, and to accurately relate them to disease status and to longitudinal patient outcome data. Only in this way will we be able to construct reliable and meaningful prediction models for oral precancer and cancer progression.

Novel therapeutic and preventive strategies   In the future, novel therapeutic and/or preventive strategies may present themselves and as clinicians we should be aware not only of scientific developments but also alert to their possible, innovative treatment roles. For example, Maley et al. have recently proposed the concept of a 'benign cell booster' cancer prevention strategy [18]. In this technique, rather than persisting with the inherently destructive concept of trying to kill (often quite indiscriminately) dysplastic or neoplastic cells in a tissue, a biological booster is introduced to increase the fitness of benign cell clones. This fascinating concept is essentially that of setting up a competitive dynamic between benign and dysplastic cells within a neoplastic field. This would adjust the ecology of the oral cavity and thus ultimately drive dysplastic cells to extinction, probably by repeated booster application over time [18].

Whether such a 'benign cell booster' actually exists and just how practical a technique it might prove to be in the clinical environment remains to be seen. However, it will probably be only through truly innovative treatment proposals such as these that further definitive progress will be made in the fight against oral carcinogenesis.

Randomised controlled trials

We have seen that many authors in the current oral precancer literature bemoan the lack of randomised controlled trials in documenting clinical outcomes in oral potentially malignant disorder patients. Holmstrup, for example, has once again recently emphasised the need for multicentre, randomised clinical trials with a long period of detailed patient follow up [19].

Despite many calls for such research to take place in the past there are very few, if any, relevant randomised trials being undertaken in oral precancer research. It is also true to say that there has never been a randomised trial comparing interventional laser surgery with either medical management or, indeed, a comparison with a control or placebo group. Why is this? Surely no researcher would dispute the scientific validity of such a trial? However, perhaps as Holmstrup observed, there are real concerns that it is potentially unethical to deny patients, particularly those with 'high-grade' dysplasia, surgical excision of their potentially malignant lesions. Similarly, if a trial was subsequently designed that excluded the perceived high-risk patients (who would presumably already be offered surgical excision) how clinically relevant would it then be to try to randomise the remaining 'low-grade' dysplasia patients into treatment or observation arms? A truly effective multicentre, randomised controlled, longitudinal follow-up study would not only be a major project but also a very expensive one. There would also have to be a clinically relevant and ethical treatment choice for patients.

The demonstrable diagnostic and treatment benefits of interventional laser surgery, which we have consistently seen in a number of our patient cohort studies, have already been heavily emphasised in this book. This is our preferred management option for potentially malignant disorders in patients who are perceived to be at high risk of malignant change. Any future clinical trial would have to add, rather than subtract, to such a treatment strategy.

What then could form the basis of a realistic, future, randomised controlled trial? Perhaps the outcomes in a laser surgery-only group could be compared with a laser-treated group combined with medical or systemic therapies? The scientific weakness of such a study remains the concern that surgical intervention itself may have a potentially deleterious influence on the natural history of oral precancer disease. Although it should be stated very clearly that we have never seen any evidence of such a hypothesis in our treated patient cohorts.

Translational research

Whilst the actual term 'translational research' may be a relatively new one, it is really only a formalisation of the classic medical research model whereby discovery and increased knowledge gained from basic scientific or laboratory research is translated into actual application in the clinical environment. This so-called 'bench to bedside' research offers a number of opportunities in oral precancer work – from the immunohistochemical studies previously described in Chapter 8 through to the application of the new scientific techniques outlined above. With the constraints inherent in trying to design randomised trials, however, it is likely that such research will be most applicable to longitudinal, observational, patient cohort studies.

Prognostic research

Generally in medicine, prognosis relates to the likelihood of an individual patient developing a particular clinical outcome over time, based upon their clinical status and/or treatment. We have discussed previously not only how important this is, but also how frustratingly difficult it can actually be in oral precancer clinical practice.

Prognostic research is thought to be best carried out as prospective, cohort studies allowing optimal measurement of predictors and outcomes although it is recognised that it may be extremely difficult to estimate study sample size. Retrospective or case–control studies and, interestingly, randomised treatment trials are actually considered less reliable for prognostic research. This is due to concerns about the overall study population, eligibility criteria and low patient recruitment and consent issues [20].

The formal development and validation of oral precancer prognosis models may in the future help improve our understanding of the determinants of both the course and clinical outcome of patients with potentially malignant disorders.

Patient experiential studies

In recent years increasing attention has been paid to encouraging the active participation of patients in biomedical research. Patients acquire specific knowledge based upon their own personal experiences of their bodies and their illnesses as well as with their care, cure and exposure to health care systems. The term 'experiential knowledge' is used to define the personal insight that arises as an individual patient learns to cope with their particular illness [21]. When patients combine their individual experiences and develop a communal body of knowledge, it is anticipated that explicit patient demands, ideas and judgements will significantly contribute to the relevance and quality of future biomedical research [21].

Interestingly, Green et al. [22] have recently undertaken a qualitative study to document the in-depth experiences of 16 oral precancer patients following their diagnosis and treatment. A number of fascinating new insights into patient views and understanding were obtained. These included misconceptions over aetiology, the impact of interventional laser treatment, the significance of the clinician–patient relationship, a number of unmet information needs, and the overall impact of a diagnosis of precancer upon their everyday lives [22].

Whilst individual and local population experiences may vary considerably, future patient experiential research is to be encouraged and may substantially add to our overall understanding of the natural history of potentially malignant disorders.

Summary

It is important for the future of oral precancer care to move forward from simply classifying patients with oral potentially malignant disorders into either high- or low-risk categories, and to strive to delineate individually tailored treatment protocols based, ideally, upon biomolecular target profiling. A variety of different treatment strategies, on occasion marshalling systemic therapies, may be appropriate for patients in differing risk categories, and both new and novel therapies should continually be sought. Better clinical outcomes will require improved response rates to interventional treatment, an enhanced immune response to premalignant disease and ultimately a reduction in the overall incidence of oral malignancy.

References

1. Hingorani AD, Shah T, Kumari M, Sofat R, Smeeth L. Translating genomics into improved healthcare. *Br Med J* 2010; 341: 1037–1042.
2. Pilling S, Yesufu-Udechuku A, Tayloe C, Drummond C. Diagnosis, assessment, and management of harmful drinking and alcohol dependence: summary of NICE guidance. *Br Med J* 2011; 342: 490–492.
3. Mehanna H, Jones TM, Gregoire V, Kian Ang K. Oropharyngeal carcinoma related to human papillomavirus. *Br Med J* 2010; 340: 879–880.
4. Hancocks S. Getting personal for a purpose. *Br Dent J* 2009; 10: 461.
5. Barbellido SA, Trapero JC, Sanchez JC, Perea Garcia MA, Castano NE, Martinez AB. Gene therapy in the management of oral cancer: review of the literature. *Med Oral Patol Oral Cir Bucal* 2008; 13: E15–E21.
6. Staples OD, Steele RJC, Lain S. p53 as a therapeutic target. *Surgeon* 2008; 6: 240–243.
7. Rudin CM, Cohen EE, Papadimitrakopoulou VA et al. An attenuated adenovirus, ONYX-015, as mouthwash therapy for premalignant oral dysplasia. *J Clin Oncol* 2003; 21: 4546–4552.
8. Price DL, Lin SF, Han Z et al. Oncolysis using herpes simplex virus type 1 engineered to express cytosine deaminase and a fusogenic glycoprotein for head and neck squamous cell carcinoma. *Arch Otolaryngol Head Neck Surg* 2010; 136: 151–158.
9. Aloysius MM, Robins RA, Eremin JM, Eremin O. Vaccination therapy in malignant disease. *The Surgeon* 2006; 4: 309–320.
10. Toomey DP, Murphy JF, Conlon KC. COX-2, VEGF and tumour angiogenesis. *The Surgeon* 2009; 7: 174–180.
11. Vokes E, Cohen E, Mauer A et al. A phase I study of erlotinib and bevacizumab for recurrent or metastatic squamous cell carcinoma of the head and neck. *J Clin Oncol* 2005; 23: 5504.
12. Goodson ML, Thomson PJ, Hamadah O. Oral dysplasia: effect of aspririn on p53 and surgical outcome. *J Dent Res* 2007; 86 (Special Issue A): 1820.
13. Hutchins GGA, Grabsch HI. Molecular pathology – the future? *The Surgeon* 2009; 7: 366–377.
14. Thompson AM. Dissecting the molecular mechanisms of human cancer: translating laboratory advances into clinical practice. *Surg J R Coll Surg Edinb Irel* 2004; 2: 1–6.
15. Shieh DB, Chou WP, Wei YH, Wong TY, Jin YT. Mitochondrial DNA 4,977-bp deletion in paired oral cancer and precancerous lesions revealed by laser microdissection and real-time quantitative PCR. *Ann N Y Acad Sci* 2004; 1011: 154–167.
16. Willeit P, Willeit J, Mayr A et al. Telomere length and risk of incident cancer and cancer mortality. *J Am Med Assoc* 2010; 304: 69–75.
17. Chuthapisith S, Layfield R, Kerr ID, Eremin O. Principles of proteomics and its application in cancer. *The Surgeon* 2007; 5: 14–22.

18. Maley CC, Reid BJ, Forrest S. Cancer prevention strategies that address the evolutionary dynamics of neoplastic cells: simulating benign cell boosters and selection for chemosensitivity. *Cancer Epidem Biomar Prev* 2004; 13: 1375–1384.

19. Holmstrup P. Can we prevent malignancy by treating premalignant lesions? *Oral Oncol* 2009; 45: 549–550.

20. Moons KGM, Royston P, Vergouwe Y, Grobbee DE, Altman DG. Prognosis and prognostic research: what, why, and how? *Br Med J* 2009; 338: 1317–1320.

21. Caron-Flinterman JF, Broerse EW, Bunders JFG. The experiential knowledge of patients: a new resource for biomedical research? *Soc Sci Med* 2005; 60: 2575–2584.

22. Green RA, Exley C, Thomson PJ, Steele JG. Understanding patient views and experience of oral precancer. *J Dent Res* 2010; 89 (Special Issue B): 2571.

11 Case Histories

Peter Thomson and Philip Sloan

Oral Precancer: Diagnosis and Management of Potentially Malignant Disorders, First Edition. Edited by Peter Thomson.
© 2012 John Wiley & Sons, Ltd. Published 2012 by John Wiley & Sons, Ltd.

Introduction

Despite its apparent simplicity, the definitive diagnosis and management of oral potentially malignant disorders remains both a complex and controversial topic for clinicians. In this chapter, therefore, we will present a number of illustrative case histories summarising the clinical presentation, histopathological diagnoses, treatment and clinical outcome for a diverse group of patients. A commentary to highlight some of the salient features of each scenario is also included. The aim of reviewing these cases is to demonstrate the principles and practice of diagnosis and clinical management, and to examine the decision-making processes expounded in the preceding chapters of this book when applied to the actual treatment of specific potentially malignant disorders of the oral mucosa.

The patient scenarios have been chosen not only to summarise common clinical presentations but also to help demonstrate some of the inherent management dilemmas seen in these clinical situations. Sometimes the decision-making process can be quite demanding and unfortunately, as we have discussed previously, there is a very limited evidence base to help guide clinicians in the treatment of many of these situations.

Case 1: diagnosis of unexpected malignancy

Clinical presentation

A 65-year-old male patient presented with a localised patch of erythroleukoplakia arising in the right anterior floor of mouth (Figure 11.1A). He had a 40-year history of tobacco smoking, usually in excess of 20 cigarettes per day, heavy and regular alcohol consumption for many years and was suffering from early-stage alcohol-related dementia when first seen. Otherwise, his medical history was relatively uncomplicated.

Histopathological diagnosis

An incisional biopsy of the floor of mouth lesion was carried out under local anaesthesia and revealed a provisional histopathological diagnosis of severe epithelial dysplasia (Figure 11.1B).

Management

In view of the presence of the severely dysplastic oral mucosa and concerns that the patient would be unlikely to stop both his smoking and his alcohol consumption, treatment comprised laser excision of the erythroleukoplakic lesion, together with a wide margin of apparently normal mucosa (Figure 11.1C). This was carried out within 2 months of his initial biopsy under general anaesthesia using the protocol described in detail in Chapter 7.

Upon histopathological examination of the excision specimen, however, a focus of superficially invasive, moderately differentiated squamous cell carcinoma was found although this had been completely excised during the laser surgery. All excision margins were reported to be free of both carcinoma and dysplasia.

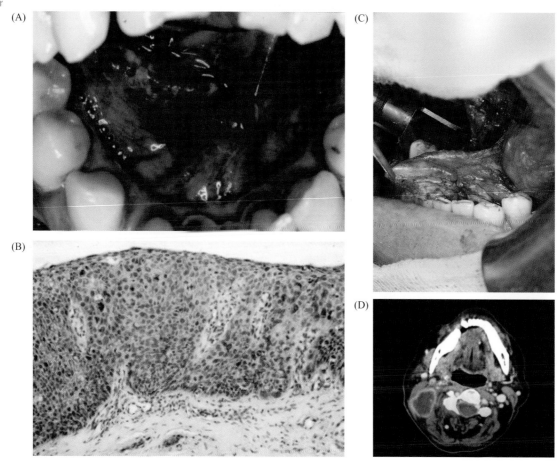

Figure 11.1 A 65-year-old male patient presenting with erythroleukoplakia in the right anterior floor of the mouth (A), provisionally diagnosed as severe dysplasia histopathologically on incisional biopsy (B). (C) Ultimately it proved to contain an early invasive squamous cell carcinoma following laser excision. (D) Fourteen months following laser surgery, a large necrotic tumour mass presented in the neck, visualised in this CT image, which also shows a smaller metastatic node situated just anterior to the sternomastoid muscle.

The patient subsequently attended the multidisciplinary head and neck cancer clinic 1 month post-laser surgery. Following clinical assessment, which confirmed no residual oral disease, and computed tomography (CT) scanning, which showed no cervical lymphadenopathy suspicious of metastatic disease, he was placed under regular monthly review and careful clinical examination.

Clinical outcome

Unfortunately, the patient only attended semi-regularly for his follow-up appointments probably as a result of his mild mental confusion, which resulted in him forgetting a number of scheduled appointments. Ultimately, at 14 months following laser surgery and after an absence from the clinic of some 4 months he re-presented, being brought back to hospital on this occasion by a concerned relative.

On clinical examination, there was a 5 cm diameter firm and fixed mass at level II in the right neck which was highly suspicious of a large deposit of metastatic carcinoma. The patient could not recall when the mass first appeared, but a visiting relative had noticed it on a domestic visit 2 weeks previously and the patient now felt it was both painful and growing rapidly in size. Intra-oral examination confirmed good healing, with minimal scarring, of the floor of the mouth at the site of the previous laser surgery and no sign could be found of any recurrent or further oral mucosal disease. Neither was there any evidence of a second primary carcinoma in the head and neck to account for the presumed metastatic lymph node disease.

Fine needle aspiration of the neck mass was carried out that confirmed the presence of squamous cell carcinoma. A CT scan of the neck was performed that visualised the large necrotic level II lymph node together with a smaller but suspiciously enlarged additional node, both of which displayed features characteristic for metastatic carcinoma. A representative image from this CT scan is shown in Figure 11.1D.

The patient subsequently underwent a radical neck dissection, which completely excised the tumour mass and confirmed the diagnosis of metastatic carcinoma with extracapsular lymph node spread around both the nodes described above, but with no other lymph node involvement. A course of adjuvant postoperative radiotherapy was applied bilaterally to the neck, and to date the patient remains well with no evidence of further disease.

Comment

It is unlikely that such a rapidly growing lymph node metastasis could have been predicted from the initial presentation of this oral lesion. Indeed, as discussed in Chapter 9, foci of unexpected carcinoma are found in approximately 10% of laser excision specimens and following their removal patients usually respond very well, attending for regular and detailed postoperative surveillance.

The site of the large necrotic node at level II was a slightly unusual presentation for an anterior floor of mouth carcinoma, which one would normally expect in the first instance to metastasise to level I submandibular lymph nodes. Nonetheless, no evidence of a synchronous primary tumour elsewhere in the head and neck region could be found, and the histological features of the neck metastasis were consistent with an origin from the initial floor of mouth lesion.

It was clearly unhelpful that the patient's mental state and social situation in this case prevented his re-attendance at clinic for several months when an earlier diagnosis of cervical lymphadenopathy may have been possible. The long-term prognosis for such a patient, of course, must remain guarded. Whilst the patient has agreed to stop smoking, there remain ongoing concerns regarding his alcohol consumption and the risks for both recurrent and further disease development.

Case 2: multiple lesion disease responding to conservative management

Clinical presentation

A 49-year-old male smoker, who had smoked approximately 15 cigarettes per day for over 30 years, presented with widespread, faint leukoplakic lesions affecting the bilateral buccal mucosae and also the dorsolateral tongue. The clinical appearance of these lesions, all of them entirely asymptomatic, is shown in Figure 11.2.

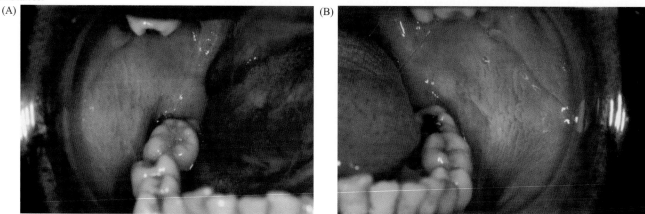

(A)   (B)

Figure 11.2   An example of widepsread, multifocal leukoplakia. There is feint leukoplakia on the right buccal mucosa (A), whilst the lesion on the left buccal mucosa exhibits a rippled or `ebbing' tide appearance (B). A small, irregular patch of dorsolateral tongue leukoplakia is also seen in (A).

Histopathological diagnosis

Incisional biopsies were taken from both buccal mucosal sites and also the dorsolateral tongue. These revealed histopathological diagnoses of hyperkeratosis at all sites, together with the presence of mild dysplasia, but this was only seen in the thickened leukoplakia arising on the left buccal mucosa.

Management

Following informed discussion, the patient undertook a period of smoking cessation counselling and, using nicotine replacement therapy, quit smoking completely by 4 weeks post diagnosis. No surgical intervention was undertaken.

Clinical outcome

The patient was followed up closely with 3-monthly review appointments arranged during the succeeding 12 months, during which time continuous improvement in the clinical appearance of the oral mucosa was observed. The patient remained a non-smoker.

A repeat incisional biopsy was taken from faint residual leukoplakia on the left buccal mucosa 18 months following the initial diagnosis. On this occasion the biopsy showed hyperkeratosis only, with no cellular atypia or any residual dysplasia evident. Further clinical improvement was noted over the next 18 months and, at approximately 3 years following initial presentation, the patient was discharged from the dysplasia clinic to the care of his general dental practitioner.

Comment

The importance of stopping smoking in improving the long-term prognosis for oral potentially malignant disorder patients cannot be overemphasised. This is especially so for multiple lesion cases in which widespread laser excisions of dysplastic mucosa may be both impractical and potentially destructive. Repeat incisional biopsies at intervals in cases that are treated by reducing risk factor behaviour and clinical observation alone are extremely useful ways of monitoring progress and, even better, demonstrating the resolution of oral potentially malignant lesions.

Case 3: multiple lesion disease requiring repeated laser treatments

Clinical presentation

A 62-year-old female smoker presented with multifocal, non-homogeneous leukoplakia arising on the right dorsolateral tongue, the floor of the mouth and mandibular alveolus (Figure 11.3A). Similar non-homogeneous lesions also affected the left posterior buccal mucosa and edentulous mandibular alveolus (Figure 11.3B). The patient reported that she smoked about 20 cigarettes per day and had done so for nearly 45 years, but consumed little in the way of alcohol.

Histopathological diagnosis

Examination under anaesthesia was undertaken and field mapping biopsies were taken from the right dorsolateral tongue, right floor of the mouth, right and left edentulous mandibular alveolar regions and left posterior buccal mucosa. Histological examination of the biopsy specimens revealed hyperkeratosis at each site but features consistent with a diagnosis of moderate dysplasia were seen in the tongue biopsy, whilst severe dysplasia was also identified in the buccal mucosa.

Management

Concerted efforts were made to encourage the patient to stop or at least reduce her smoking. Laser excisions of the right dorsolateral tongue leukoplakia and the left posterior buccal mucosa leukoplakia were undertaken.

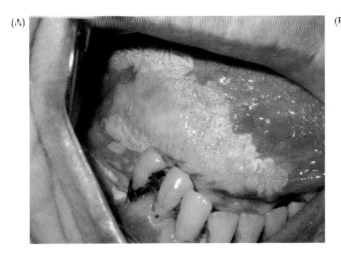
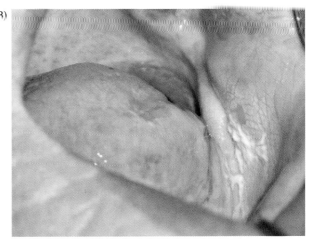

Figure 11.3 In this example of multiple lesion disease, there is widespread non-homogeneous leukoplakia affecting the right dorsolateral tongue, floor of the mouth and mandibular alveolus (A), whilst further non-homogeneous leukoplakia appears on the left buccal mucosa (B).

Clinical outcome

Complete resolution of the left buccal mucosa disease was seen but unfortunately the patient continued to smoke, albeit at a reduced number of cigarettes per day. Residual disease was observed on the right posterolateral tongue 6 weeks following laser treatment and further laser surgery was arranged to excise this lesion 4 months later. Clinical resolution occurred subsequent to this further surgery, but at 2 years follow up a recurrent patch of leukoplakia was observed arising at a more anterior location on the right lateral tongue. Incisional biopsy confirmed moderate dysplasia at this site and thus a third laser excision was carried out to remove this lesion.

Since then, the patient has remained free of lesions on the lateral tongue, whilst the leukoplakia seen originally at the floor of mouth and mandibular alveolar sites has remained although this is asymptomatic and has reduced in both lesion extent and thickness.

Comment

Repeated laser treatments are sometimes required, especially in cases with widespread multifocal disease. Patients usually tolerate multiple treatments well, scarring is not usually a problem and ultimately clinical resolution may be achieved. Long-term follow up is, of course, mandatory and, ideally, improved risk factor behaviour should be attempted.

Case 4: proliferative verrucous leukoplakia

Clinical presentation

A 45-year-old male patient presented who complained of an 'uncomfortable and roughened patch of gum' affecting his left mandibular buccal gingiva in the premolar and molar regions. He also reported intermittent soreness of his gingiva at various other oral sites. The patient was a non-smoker, consumed less than 5 units of alcohol per week and was generally fit and well.

Clinical examination revealed a linear, raised patch of proliferative verrucous leukoplakia (PVL) extending from the first premolar to the second molar tooth and affecting both the marginal and attached buccal gingivae (Figure 11.4A). There were also lichenoid lesions affecting the right posterior maxillary buccal gingiva and the adjacent buccal mucosa together with a localised verrucous leukoplakic patch affecting the right anterior maxillary gingiva.

Histopathological diagnosis

Incisional biopsies were taken under local anaesthesia from both the mandibular leukoplakic gingival lesion and the maxillary buccal gingiva. The lesions had common histopathological appearances, specifically the appearance of verrucous hyperplasia and lichenoid inflammatory change in the subjacent connective tissue. In addition, mild epithelial dysplasia was observed in the left mandibular gingiva specimen. A provisional diagnosis of PVL was thus made.

Management

A detailed examination of the entire oral cavity and oropharynx was carried out under general anaesthesia, although no additional mucosal lesions were

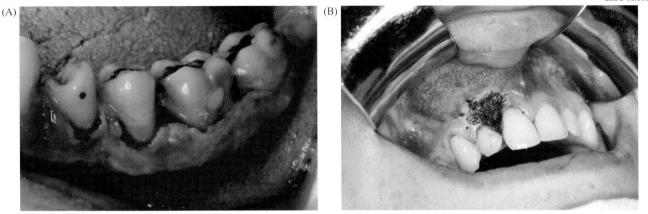

Figure 11.4 (A) An example of proliferative verrucous leukoplakia arising on the mandibular buccal gingival. (B) Following laser ablation of a more localised verrucous lesion on the maxillary gingiva.

identified. Immediately following this, laser ablation of the left mandibular gingival lesion and the right maxillary anterior gingiva was carried out using the surgical technique described in Chapter 7. Figure 11.4B demonstrates the post-laser ablation appearance of the maxillary gingiva. The patient was subsequently followed up in the dysplasia clinic.

Clinical outcome

Excellent gingival healing with minimal scarring was noted post laser with no residual leukoplakia. During the initial postoperative follow up there were no changes in any of the lichenoid lesions. Unfortunately, at about 10 months following laser treatment, the patient noticed recurrence of a small, white, roughened patch of gingiva just apical to the site of his previous surgery. Recurrence of the PVL was therefore diagnosed, but to date this has remained both localised and asymptomatic so no further surgical intervention has been deemed necessary. The patient remains under regular dysplasia clinic follow up.

Comment

As we discussed in Chapter 4, the recognition and specific diagnosis of PVL has important implications for long-term patient management. With a reported malignant transformation rate as high as 70%, interventional treatment is definitely recommended, but the high rate of subsequent lesion recurrence makes regular and consistent clinical follow up mandatory in patient management.

Formal laser excision of gingival lesions, which is normally advocated for dysplastic lesions at other oral sites, is impractical owing to the resultant dehiscence of the underlying alveolar bone, slow protracted healing and ultimately poor aesthetics. Whilst laser ablation is thus a pragmatic alternative and also highly acceptable to patients, it does unfortunately increase the likelihood of lesion recurrence due to the retention of intact mucoperiosteal tissue.

Review of a number of recently treated PVL lesions reveals definite clinical and histopathological similarities between PVL and lesions with significant lichenoid features. It seems quite clear that all mucosal lesions apparently falling in to these clinical categories should have incisional biopsies to delineate provisional histological diagnoses. The correlation of histological and clinical appearances is an important part of diagnosis.

Case 5: localised oral lichenoid reaction

Clinical presentation

A 50-year-old female patient presented with a painful, erosive lesion on the right buccal mucosa which was causing her both intermittent pain and localised sensitivity. The patient was a non-smoker and rarely consumed alcohol, and was otherwise fit and well. Clinical examination confirmed a well localised, erosive, lichenoid lesion immediately adjacent to an old corroded amalgam restoration in a mandibular molar tooth (Figure 11.5). There was no history of skin irritation, nor were any cutaneous lesions seen on examination.

Histopathological diagnosis

A local anaesthetic incisional biopsy was carried out that revealed an atrophic epithelium, together with liquefactive degeneration of the basal cells and a well-defined band of lymphocytes and histiocytes in the immediately subjacent connective tissue. This was consistent with a diagnosis of a lichenoid reaction, probably secondary to a mercury salt hypersensitivity and local frictional trauma. The epithelium, however, was also reported as exhibiting changes consistent with moderate dysplasia.

Management

In view of the presence of dysplasia, and the absence of obvious aetiological agents such as tobacco and alcohol consumption, a decision was made to formally excise the lichenoid lesion by laser under general anaesthesia. This was carried out 1 month after the incision biopsy and subsequent histopathological examination confirmed the provisional diagnosis of a moderately dysplastic lichenoid lesion. The lesion was completely excised, and all margins were reported as free of dysplastic change.

In addition, the patient attended her general dental practitioner who coordinated smoothing of the buccal cusps of the molar tooth and replacement of the amalgam with a composite resin restoration to try to avoid further local mucosal irritation.

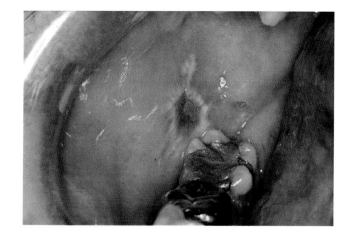

Figure 11.5 Localised oral lichenoid reaction, adjacent to an old amalgam restoration. Histopathological examination revealed moderate dysplasia within the epithelium and as a consequence the lesion was excised by laser and the amalgam replaced.

Clinical outcome

To date the patient has remained well, with no sign of lesion recurrence or further lichenoid eruptions intra-orally. Gradually, over the ensuing months, the patient had all her remaining amalgam restorations either removed and replaced by composites or covered by coronal restorations.

Comment

Oral mucosal lichenoid changes adjacent to old, often large, amalgam restorations are a particularly common clinical presentation. It is recommended that all such lesions are biopsied, not only to confirm the clinical diagnosis but to look for the presence of epithelial dysplasia. Anecdotally, as we discussed in Chapter 4, such lichenoid dysplastic lesions are inherently unstable and often proceed to carcinoma development in the absence of classic tobacco and alcohol aetiological agents. Their complete excision is thus advised. Similarly, even in the absence of frank dysplasia on biopsy, it is deemed appropriate to replace or cover amalgam restorations in these patients to prevent further mucosal irritation. The mucosal response can then be carefully monitored to ensure complete lesion resolution.

Single, localised, lichenoid lesions are relatively straightforward to manage in the manner discussed above. A more taxing clinical management problem arises, however, when multiple lichenoid lesions become more widespread, affecting numerous, distinct intra-oral sites.

Case 6: multiple oral lichenoid reactions

Clinical presentation

In this presentation a 53-year-old non-smoking female patient displayed widespread and painful, erosive, lichenoid lesions. These were distributed bilaterally on the buccal mucosa but were especially concentrated around old, large amalgam restorations in her posterior molar teeth (Figure 11.6).

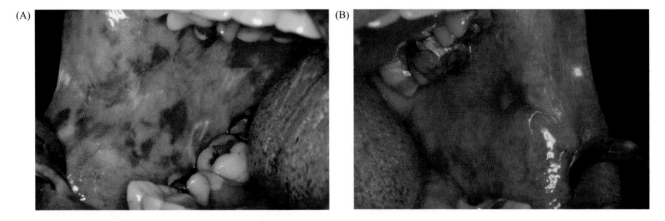

Figure 11.6 Widespread oral lichenoid reactions affecting both the right (A) and left (B) buccal mucosae, with the mucosal lesions concentrated around old amalgam restorations, particularly in the molar teeth.

Histopathological diagnosis

In view of the bilateral presentation, local anaesthetic incisional biopsies of both the right and left buccal lesions were carried out. These confirmed the clinical impression of probable lichenoid reactions to amalgam. Mild dysplasia was seen in the left buccal lesion (Figure 11.6B), whilst reactive atypia only was observed in the right buccal mucosa.

Management

Arrangements were made to remove and replace all the old amalgam restorations and the patient underwent laser excision of the lichenoid lesion arising at the left labio-buccal site. Histopathological examination of the excision specimen showed widespread dysplasia up to moderate grade throughout the excision specimen, with foci of mild dysplasia present at the excision margins.

Clinical outcome

Healing took place uneventfully following laser treatment and, subsequent to amalgam restoration replacement, the oral mucosa returned to a normal appearance with no further lesions or mucosal sensitivity. The patient remains under long-term follow up in the dysplasia clinic.

Comment

The presence of multiple oral lesions always poses a difficult management problem, particularly in regard to just how much surgical intervention is warranted and over what time scale it should be carried out. The best guide to directing interventional treatment remains the use of field mapping biopsies. We therefore recommend multiple, incisional biopsies in all such cases to determine both the range and extent of dysplastic change in a widespread mucosal abnormality. Targeting the most significantly dysplastic areas with surgery, followed by active and coordinated follow up, remains the most efficacious treatment strategy for such cases.

It is probably not surprising that some dysplastic foci are found in excision margins in lesions excised from multiple or pan-oral dysplasia cases. It is highly likely that large areas of clinically normal-looking mucosa in such patients already harbour regions of pre-existing but clinically undetectable dysplasia.

The fact that all laser excision procedures also involve the use of de-focused laser beam vapourisation, which effectively extends treatment beyond the excision margins into adjacent mucosa, is thus a particularly beneficial feature of carbon dioxide laser function.

Case 7: widespread dysplastic oral lichenoid lesions

Clinical presentation

In this clinical scenario, which did not relate to any specific association with amalgam restorative material or to any identifiable drug reaction, a 40-year-old non-smoking patient presented with painful, bilateral, roughened patches on

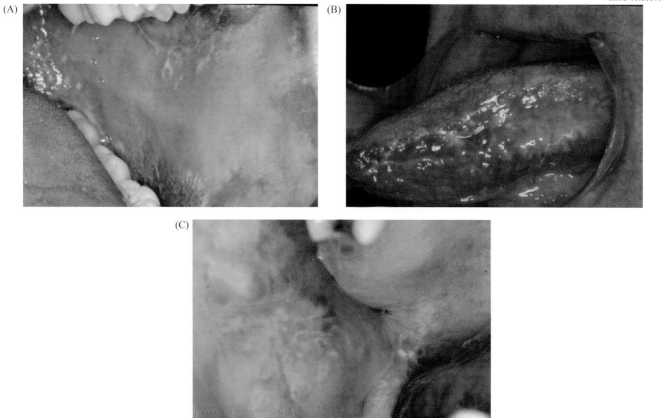

(A) (B) (C)

Figure 11.7 Multifocal dysplastic oral lichenoid lesions affecting the left buccal mucosa (A) and lateral tongue (B) in a widespread pattern. (C) A more localised presentation is seen arising on the right buccal mucosa.

both her buccal mucosa and her tongue. The clinical appearance of these widespread lichenoid lesions is shown in Figure 11.7. There was no history of cutaneous lesions, and the patient was otherwise fit and well.

Histopathological diagnosis

In view of the widespread presentation, field mapping biopsies were carried out from the upper and lower left buccal lesions, the left lateral tongue and the right buccal mucosa. All lesions exhibited significant lichenoid features on histopathological examination. However, the upper buccal lesion on the left side and the right buccal mucosa lesion both demonstrated features consistent with mild to moderate dysplasia.

Management

Laser excisions were carried out of the upper left buccal mucosal lesion (Figure 11.7A) and the right mid-buccal mucosal lesion (Figure 11.7C). Histopathological examination of the excision specimens confirmed the provisional diagnosis of moderate dysplasia, which was deemed to have been completely excised at both sites.

Clinical outcome

Good healing took place at both buccal mucosa laser sites, with minimal scarring. However, lichenoid lesions persisted on the buccal and lingual mucosae at untreated sites. A further biopsy was taken from the persistent lower left buccal lesion 18 months later which showed hyperkeratosis and lichenoid inflammation only with no evidence of dysplasia. To date, the patient remains well with no evidence of further dysplasia development.

Comment

Whilst lichen planus and lichenoid lesions are common clinical presentations, it is much less common to identify widespread dysplasia in such cases. However, in our experience, certain patients do present with dysplastic lichenoid lesions and this appears to predispose to a higher risk of malignant transformation. Like all multiple lesion cases, these risks are increased when large areas of oral mucosa are affected. Many patients affected by dysplastic lichenoid lesions are young, fit and healthy, are often female and are rarely smokers. This particular type of clinical presentation should be regarded as a high-risk case because of the increased likelihood of squamous cell carcinoma development.

Follow up of such patients, in whom some mucosal lesions have been excised but where large areas of clinically abnormal mucosa remain, is very difficult. It is impossible to say, for example, that the patient has no residual disease following treatment, because clinical examination invariably confirms the presence of persistent lesions. Meanwhile, the monitoring of patients and their re-examinations can be confusing due to post-laser scarring occurring amidst residual clinical disease.

It is precisely in these cases where diagnostic adjuncts, as described in Chapter 4, are so helpful in both imaging and analysing widespread, abnormal mucosal fields. The timing and selection of oral sites for further biopsy remains highly subjective, requiring both experience in the clinical management of oral dysplasia and a detailed knowledge of the individual patient's potentially malignant disorder and clinical course.

Case 8: an immunosuppressed patient

Clinical presentation

This case involved a 70-year-old male patient who had undergone a renal transplant 8 years prior to presenting with facial skin lesions, dryness and crusting of his lower lip and soreness at the angles of his mouth. Clinical examination revealed the presence of a cutaneous squamous cell carcinoma on the right nasal bridge near the medial canthus of the eye (Figure 11.8A) together with lichenoid-looking lesions on the lower labial mucosa (Figure 11.8B). Erythroleukoplakia was also seen arising at both labial commissures, but with a more extensive presentation on the left side.

Histopathological diagnosis

Excision biopsy of the localised facial skin lesion was carried out confirming complete excision of a well-differentiated squamous cell carcinoma. Incisional

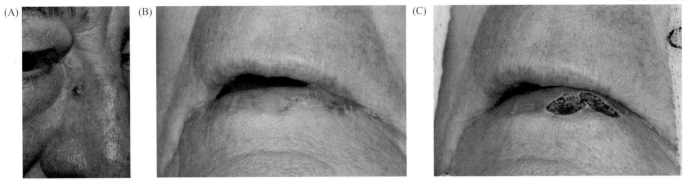

(A)   (B)   (C)

Figure 11.8 A 70-year-old post-renal transplant patient exhibiting squamous cell carcinoma on the facial skin (A), together with mild dysplasia arising on the lower left labial mucosa (B). (C) The skin carcinoma was excised and the labial mucosal lesion treated by laser ablation therapy.

biopsies were also taken from the labial mucosa and both commissures revealing mildly dysplastic features at all sites.

Management

In relation to the lip and labial commissures, laser ablation was applied to the labial mucosa (Figure 11.8C), whilst small localised laser excisions were carried out to excise the dysplastic labial commissure lesions.

Clinical outcome

Initial healing was excellent at all sites. Over the ensuing 3 years, the patient developed two further facial skin lesions, an actinic keratosis and an early invasive squamous cell carcinoma, which were both ultimately excised. A further laser excision was required to remove recurrent leukoplakia at the left labial commissure.

Comment

As one of the commonest potentially malignant conditions, immunosuppression can give rise to a number of facial skin and oral mucosal lesions, both synchronously and metachronously. Careful, regular and repeated clinical follow up and examination are required long term for such patients.

Case 9: chronic hyperplastic candidosis

Clinical presentation

A 44-year-old male patient was referred by his general dental practitioner regarding feint, irregular leukoplakic patches in the labial commissure regions bilaterally and also the lower left labial mucosa. The clinical appearance of these lesions are shown in Figure 11.9. The patient was an insulin-dependent diabetic and had smoked approximately 20 cigarettes per day for 20 years, but was otherwise fit and well.

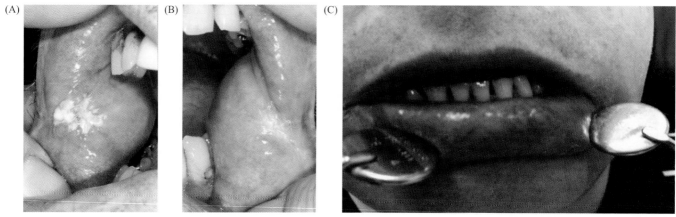

Figure 11.9 Chronic hyperplastic candidosis presenting as thickened, non-homogeneous leukoplakia on the right labial commissure (A) and as feint leukoplakia on the left labial commissure (B). (C) A further feint eryrthroleukoplakic lesion is seen on the lower labial mucosa.

Histopathological diagnosis

A local anaesthetic incision biopsy was taken from the lesion arising on the right labial commissure as this was the most clinically distinct lesion (Figure 11.9A). Features of hyperkeratosis, prominent irregular acanthosis combined with oedema and superficial microabscess formation, and invasion of the parakeratin by candidal pseudohyphae confirmed the histopathological diagnosis as a chronic hyperplastic candidosis. Moderate dysplasia was present in the epithelium.

Management

Initial management comprised smoking cessation advice and systemic antifungal medication using the orally administered triazole drug fluconazole, 50 mg daily for 14 days. Unfortunately, the patient continued to smoke and all three lesions persisted with little change in appearance. At 3 months post-fluconazole treatment, therefore, and in view of the presence of moderate dysplasia in the initial incisional biopsy, both labial commissure lesions were excised by laser (see Chapter 7). The labial mucosa lesion (Figure 11.9C) was ablated rather than excised in order to preserve the appearance of the lower lip.

Histopathological examination of both labial commissure excision specimens supported the provisional diagnosis of chronic hyperplastic candidosis, and the presence of moderate epithelial dysplasia was confirmed at both sites. All excision margins, however, were free of dysplastic change.

Clinical outcome

All laser-treated sites healed well with minimal scarring only and no residual disease and no recurrent or further lesions were seen during 2 years of subsequent follow up. Despite several attempts at smoking cessation, however, the patient unfortunately continued to smoke on an intermittent basis throughout this period.

Comment

Although sometimes single, the lesions of chronic hyperplastic candidosis are most frequently bilateral and often contain foci of epithelial dysplasia. Whilst antifungal therapy and attempts to stop patients smoking should always form the first line of management, it is our experience that labial commissure lesions usually persist indefinitely, often slowly worsening in clinical appearance, until they are formally excised.

As at other oral sites, laser surgery facilitates complete lesion removal with both excellent healing and minimal scarring. At the commissure region, it is also possible to extend the excision past the vermilion border onto skin if required, still preserving a good cosmetic appearance.

There remains, of course, a small risk of both lesion recurrence and new lesion development in patients who continue to smoke and all cases should be followed up and examined regularly.

Case 10: tobacco-associated hyperkeratosis

Clinical presentation

A 29-year-old male postgraduate student newly arrived in the UK from the Sudan attended for a routine check up at the university dental service. He had never previously accessed dental care. A folded, painless, white lesion involving the oral vestibule, gingival margin and labial mucosa in the upper left central and lateral incisor region was noted on intra-oral examination (Figure 11.10). The patient was not aware of having a lesion and consequently its duration was unknown. There was no cervical lymphadenopathy and no other abnormal findings were apparent on intra-oral or extra-oral examination. The patient was a non-smoker and drank no alcohol. No significant medical history was noted and the patient could offer no explanation for the lesion. He denied any relevant habits, including the use of topical agents or medications in that area of the mouth. The patient was advised to have an incisional biopsy of the white patch for further assessment and also to return for routine periodontal treatment at a later time.

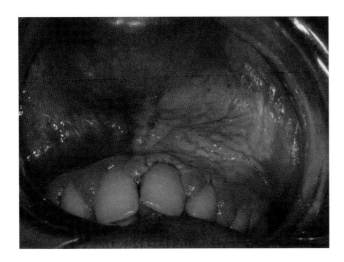

Figure 11.10 Toombak-associated hyperkeratosis. This Sudanese postgraduate student presented with a discrete folded hyperkeratotic white lesion in the upper left labial vestibule.

Histopathological diagnosis

The incisional biopsy showed an oral mucosa that exhibited acanthosis and folded hyperparakeratosis. The surface layers of the oral epithelium were pale staining and the lamina propria contained dense eosinophilic hyaline collagen. There was basal cell hyperplasia but cytological atypia was minimal and in keeping with reactive changes. The overall maturation pattern of the epithelium was preserved and only scattered inflammatory cells were present in the lamina propria. The basement membrane was prominent. A diagnosis of mild dysplasia was suggested by the original reporting pathologist and the patient was referred for a specialist opinion. Review of the biopsy was also requested.

Management

At the specialist oral medicine clinic the patient continued to deny using any oral substances, but when asked specifically about the use of toombak he admitted that he did regularly place this in the vestibule at the site of the lesion, but as he had done so since he was 12 years old he did not think it was worth mentioning! Review of the histopathology slides was undertaken by two consultant oral and maxillofacial pathologists. It was agreed that the changes could be explained by a reactive process to toombak use and that the degree of cytological atypia was actually insufficient for a diagnosis of dysplasia.

Clinical outcome

The patient was informed about the risks of using toombak and management options were explored including possible laser removal of the lesion. The patient felt that he could quit his long habit of using toombak and expressed a strong preference for 'watchful waiting'. Fortunately the patient was compliant and the lesion gradually reduced over a 3-month period and the mucosa was completely normal clinically after 1 year. The patient was followed for 2 further years with no recurrence of the lesion, after which he returned to the Sudan.

Comment

We have seen already that on a global basis oral potentially malignant lesions can be associated with a variety of tobacco products used in a number of different ways in the oral cavity. The link with oral cancer, however, is often not known to the users, as indeed was the case for this patient. Toombak is a form of moist chewing tobacco manufactured in the Sudan. It has one of the highest contents of un-ionised nicotine and carcinogenic tobacco-specific N-nitrosamines of all such tobacco products. The recorded incidence of epithelial dysplasia in toombak-related lesions is low, however, and it is likely that many of the clinically keratotic lesions result from chemical injury.

Nevertheless the incidence of oral cancer in Sudan is high and use of toombak is clearly risky. In the present case the complete resolution of the lesion provides evidence of its reactive nature. Also in this instance, awareness of the tobacco products that are likely to be used in particular regions helped to prompt and elicit a critical part of the history. Fortunately the patient was highly intelligent, single minded and health conscious and was able to quit the habit. However, oral tobacco products can actually be more difficult to quit than smoking, and all available cessation methods should always be offered to patients who use chewing tobaccos.

Case 11: malignant transformation in longstanding non-erosive lichen planus

Clinical presentation and history

A male patient aged 34 years had been referred to a hospital department of oral medicine with a diagnosis of oral lichen planus. He had noticed that his tongue had looked white for some time but was otherwise symptomless (Figure 11.11A). The referral was only made when he attended his dental practitioner for a routine check up who also noted bilateral buccal mucosal white patches. The appearance of the patient's right and left buccal mucosa at this time is shown in Figure 11.11B and C.

The patient reported that he had been a light, social smoker between the ages of 17 and 26 years but had given up when his father was diagnosed with lung cancer. His alcohol intake was 7 units per week and his medical history was otherwise unremarkable.

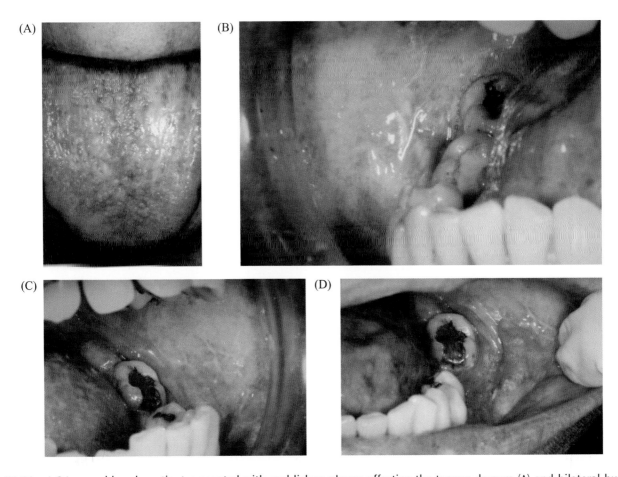

Figure 11.11 A 34-year-old male patient presented with oral lichen planus affecting the tongue dorsum (A) and bilateral buccal mucosa (B, C). (D) The thickened, irregular, left buccal mucosa on re-presentation 8 years later. Biopsy of this latter lesion showed squamous cell carcinoma.

An incisional biopsy of the left buccal mucosa taken at the hospital at this time showed features of hyperkeratosis with lichenoid inflammation, in keeping with the clinical diagnosis of lichen planus. No treatment was prescribed. The patient was followed up for 2 years and then discharged back to the care of his dentist.

He attended regular dental appointments and oral inspections until 8 years after the original referral when the dentist referred him back to hospital because he had detected a palpably firm area in the left buccal mucosa. This lesion, which was asymptomatic and only conspicuous on careful clinical examination, is illustrated in Figure 11.11D. The patient's dental practitioner, however, was certain that this lesion had not been present 6 months previously.

Histopathological diagnosis

Following re-attendance at the hospital clinic, an incisional biopsy of the buccal lesion was carried out that showed the presence of a moderately differentiated invasive squamous cell carcinoma arising at this site. The initial incisional biopsy from 8 years previously was therefore reviewed and confirmed squamous mucosa with acanthosis, hyperparakeratosis and a subepithelial band of lymphohistiocytic infiltrate. Lymphocyte exocytosis was present and there was basal cell liquefaction degeneration. Civatte bodies were also present. The biopsy was viewed independently by two oral and maxillofacial pathologists, neither of whom found any evidence of epithelial dysplasia. Both pathologists thus agreed with the original diagnosis of a hyperkeratosis with lichenoid inflammation.

Management

Clinical examination and CT scanning confirmed that this was a stage I tumour, with no evidence of extensive local invasion or cervical lymph node involvement. The carcinoma was thus removed by laser excision. Histopathological examination of the excised specimen revealed the presence of a discrete, moderately differentiated, squamous cell carcinoma, measuring 1.6 mm in diameter and 2.3 mm maximum thickness, which had been completely excised.

Clinical outcome

Postoperative healing proceeded well during the immediate follow-up period but at 5 months following the buccal excision an enlarged, firm, cervical lymph node appeared in the ipsilateral neck at level II. CT scanning and fine needle aspiration cytology confirmed metastatic squamous carcinoma and as a result a modified left radical neck dissection was performed.

Histopathological examination of the neck dissection specimen showed a 22 mm deposit of squamous cell carcinoma with extracapsular spread at level II, whilst a further eight nodes containing metastatic carcinoma were found distributed between levels I, II and IV. As a result of this extensive nodal involvement, postoperative radiotherapy was administered but, unfortunately, the tumour recurred both locally in the buccal tissues and in the neck and the patient died 1 year after his final treatment.

Comment

This case raises a number of both interesting and difficult questions. As we discussed in Chapter 4, there is still no consensus as to whether lichen planus should be regarded as a truly potentially malignant oral lesion or not.

This patient had been exposed to risk factors, but not to an excessive extent, and was still relatively young. He was not therefore considered to fall into the category of oral carcinoma development linked to the ongoing use of tobacco and alcohol, with a coincidental diagnosis of lichen planus. On the contrary, this tumour presentation appeared to take place as a result of the direct transformation of a previously identified lichenoid precursor into an invasive carcinoma.

Whilst established buccal carcinomas can exhibit significant local invasion and may prove difficult to manage, the small carcinoma identified in this case showed an unusually aggressive biological behaviour, despite effective surgical excision, ultimately leading to a rapidly progressing poor clinical outcome. Such phenomena have indeed been previously linked to carcinomas arising in longstanding lichen planus in a number of anecdotal reports. As yet, however, no published series provides convincing evidence to help explain the particularly aggressive behaviour of carcinomas that develop from lichenoid lesions, but one must consider that aberrant immunological factors are likely to be involved.

This case also raises concerns regarding the efficacy of follow-up protocols for patients diagnosed with oral lichen planus and lichenoid lesions. It is impractical to suggest that all such patients should remain under specialist care, especially when they attend their general dental practitioners for routine oral inspections. However, the question remains how can we possibly recognise those patients that may be at high risk of malignant transformation or cancer development and who thus require more intensive and specialist care?

Undoubtedly, the oral dysplasia clinic offers optimal opportunities for diagnosis, review and intervention for potentially malignant lesions but, as seen in the case above, many lichenoid lesions that transform to carcinoma did not demonstrate any dysplastic features on incisional biopsy. Similarly, there are no clear guidelines as to how often biopsies should be taken for histopathological re-examination of clinical lesions during follow up. Multiple, repeated biopsy sampling is unpopular with patients and indeed such repeated surgical interventions within a persistent lesion may even be potentially harmful to unstable mucosal lesions.

It seems unlikely that any alternative or additional clinical intervention could have altered the unfortunate course of this patient's disease. It remains the ultimate frustration and failure of potentially malignant disorder management to report the malignant transformation and ultimate death of a patient who presented with an identifiable oral precursor lesion.

Summary

In this chapter we have reviewed 11 case histories in which the diagnosis and management of patients presenting with a variety of oral potentially malignant disorders have been presented and discussed. It is hoped that these practical examples help to demonstrate both the rationale for, and also some of the inherent difficulties that remain within, the decision-making process described in this book. It is very important to note that, despite specialist diagnosis and interventional management, we are not always able to halt the potentially lethal process of oral carcinogenesis. Every potentially malignant disorder patient must therefore be considered 'at risk' of oral cancer and we must continue our efforts to obtain more accurate risk stratification, improve our ability to tailor treatment programmes more individually to patients, and to develop clinically applicable predictive tools to determine clinical outcome.

12 Conclusions

Peter Thomson

Oral Precancer: Diagnosis and Management of Potentially Malignant Disorders, First Edition. Edited by Peter Thomson.
© 2012 John Wiley & Sons, Ltd. Published 2012 by John Wiley & Sons, Ltd.

Oral cancer

Oral squamous cell carcinoma is a lethal and deforming disease and, as we have seen, there is a serious and realistic threat that a global epidemic of mouth cancer may occur during the 21st century. The last few decades have seen real advances in diagnostic techniques, refinements in ablative tumour surgery and improvements in complex surgical reconstruction of the mouth and face. All of these developments, together with modern chemoradiotherapy regimes, have undoubtedly improved the loco-regional control and quality of life for oral cancer patients.

Unfortunately, however, 5-year mortality rates remain at near 50% levels with patients still dying from local recurrence and now increasingly from widespread blood-borne metastases as well. It has also been recognised more recently that second or even third primary tumours may affect patients as a result of field change cancerisation in the upper aerodigestive tract, and that such recalcitrant disease is highly likely to ultimately prove fatal.

Any further improvements in the mortality rates for mouth cancer will thus require much earlier intervention during the process of carcinogenesis. The oral cavity, unlike many other high-risk upper aerodigestive tract sites, is readily inspected. We are also fortunate to recognise that many, if not all, oral cancers are preceded by pre-invasive potentially malignant disorders that can be detected as either localised or sometimes more widespread mucosal abnormalities.

Potentially malignant disorders

Potentially malignant disorders may thus present as localised intra-oral leukoplakias, erythroplakias and mixed erythroleukoplakic lesions, and sometimes as more widespread mucosal conditions or as manifestations of systemic conditions. All of these share a common but unpredictable propensity for cancer development.

Whilst the clinical recognition of a mucosal abnormality is relatively straightforward, the precise diagnosis ascribed to an individual patient presenting with a potentially malignant disorder is in reality a more demanding process, which requires detailed coordination of specific clinical and pathological data. More recently, we have recognised the importance and desirability of being able to distinguish 'high-risk' from 'low-risk' cases, in terms of the overall likelihood of transformation to malignancy.

Historically, there has been confusion and disagreement over both the appropriateness and the effectiveness of treatment for oral potentially malignant disorders. In this book we have presented a case for a proactive and interventional management strategy based upon laser surgical excision of individual potentially malignant lesions and a careful and detailed post-surgical follow up and oral surveillance.

Clinical management

Interventional surgical treatment, as illustrated in practice in the operating theatre in Figure 12.1, is effective in removing active precancer disease, and thus

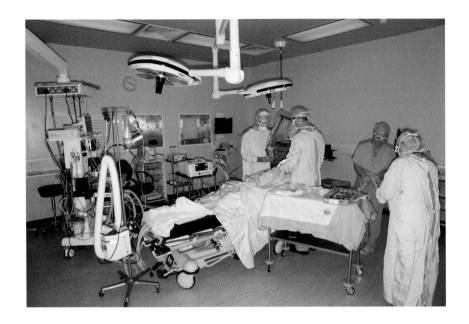

Figure 12.1 Interventional intra-oral laser surgery in progress in the operating theatre.

preventing same-site malignant transformation in nearly two-thirds of patients. It also facilitates definitive diagnosis of lesions, and in clinical practice has been shown to be able to identify and excise pre-existing, clinically undetectable squamous carcinoma in approximately 10% of all treated oral precancer patients. It seems very difficult, therefore, to support alternative management strategies based upon observational or medical treatments that do not offer such comprehensive opportunities for definitive histopathological diagnosis and efficacious treatment. These comments apply not only to identifiable potentially malignant lesions, but also to those cases of early invasive cancer of the oral mucosa that would have otherwise remained hidden until a much later stage of clinical presentation.

The patient subgroups that demand further intensive study and investigation are those in the remaining one-third of cases in which precancer disease may unfortunately persist, recur or develop into further lesions at new oral sites following laser excision. It is presumed that it is within these particular groups that precancer disease is at its most aggressive and unstable, and it is also likely to be these patients who are at the greatest risk of malignant transformation occurring.

Whether the biological nature of oral potentially malignant disorders truly varies between disease-free and recurrent or further disease patients or between single lesion and multiple lesion presentation – or is actually more of a reflection of disease severity or progression at a particular moment in time in an individual patient – remains to be seen. We have, however, demonstrated real clinical and pathological differences in these differing patient groups in our clinic studies and such observations have undoubtedly had a clear practical application in developing appropriately tailored management strategies.

The ultimate aim in the diagnosis and management of oral potentially malignant disorders must be the prevention of oral cancer. We believe that we have clearly demonstrated that the risk of malignant transformation, or same-site cancer development, can indeed be reduced by formal excision of precancer tissue. At the same time we recognise that 'high-risk' patients may still go on to develop carcinoma at new, distinct intra-oral sites and that this remains highly unpredictable.

209

Patient care pathways

Central to the diagnosis and management of potentially malignant disorders is, undeniably, the overall care pathways we provide for our patients. In this book, we have proposed and explained the benefits of a structured and coordinated interventional management strategy. We have also seen very clearly that, due to the unpredictable risk of metachronous precancer or cancer disease development, all oral precancer patients, irrespective of their initial presenting disease and treatment outcomes, should be carefully followed up long term. The opportunity to continually reinforce the benefits of reducing harmful risk factor behaviour and the ability to carry out mucosal surveillance for recurrent or further oral lesions thereby facilitates both risk reduction and early diagnosis of disease.

There are inevitably health care costs associated with long-term follow up of patients, but this is relatively inconsequential compared to the financial burden associated with the treatment of established head and neck malignancy. We strongly believe that the ideal environment for managing precancer patients is in dedicated, specialist oral potentially malignant disorder or dysplasia clinics. Within such a service, a multidisciplinary clinical team approach is desirable. The essential components of a potentially malignant disorder clinical service are summarised in Box 12.1.

Box 12.1 Essential components of a clinical service for potentially malignant disorders.

Clinical team
- Lead clinician: oral and maxillofacial surgeon and/or oral physician
- Dedicated and regular nursing staff in attendance
- Smoking cessation therapist

Clinical facilities
- Dedicated weekly clinic for new referrals and follow-up cases
- Immediately accessible biopsy service
- Full range of available diagnostic adjuncts
- Regular access to in-patient operating facilities
- Carbon dioxide laser surgery

Support services
- Specialist oral and maxillofacial pathology services
- Experienced oral cytology service
- Anaesthetic support specialised in intra-oral laser surgery
- Medical physics support for carbon dioxide laser services
- Head and neck radiology and imaging services
- Medical photography

Access
- Access to multidisciplinary head and neck cancer team

The importance of a consistent approach and the availability of the same clinical team to attend patients cannot be overemphasised, not only in terms of the overall quality of clinical care but also in relation to patient involvement, engagement and acceptance of that care. Such care is, of course, fundamental not only to interventional treatment but even more so for effective preventive strategies.

It is unfortunate however that, despite an ongoing programme of active research work, we still lack the ability to predict clinical outcome and disease progression for any patient who presents with a potentially malignant oral disorder. This is a real frustration for both clinicians and patients themselves. Nonetheless, observational clinical behaviour data have been obtained from our several patient cohort studies which can help plan follow-up care to some extent. For example, those patients with milder disease who stop smoking and are disease-free for 3 years post treatment may be safely followed up by their general dental practitioner. This presupposes that the patient has their own dentist and that they do indeed attend for regular 6-monthly check ups. In contrast, patients with more severe dysplastic disease, multiple lesion presentation or in whom precancer exists in the absence of obvious exposure to harmful risk factors are undoubtedly better followed up in the dysplasia clinic environment.

Public health strategies

All of the above patient-centred care provides a pragmatic and reasonably successful strategy for managing those patients who present to clinicians with identifiable oral precancers. However, there remains the much wider problem that the majority of patients with high-risk factor behaviour rarely, if ever, attend for regular oral examination, advice or treatment. More widespread oral cancer and precancer preventive strategies will thus become increasingly important in the years ahead, as will attempts to identify and target high-risk individuals or specific patient groups at enhanced risk of oral cancer to facilitate early diagnosis and intervention on a population-wide basis.

Future directions

We have already discussed in some detail a number of possible future developments in the diagnosis and management of oral precancer (see Chapter 10). Suffice to say again here that the future will undoubtedly see rapid developments in biomolecular medicine and, ultimately, it is hoped that the tailoring of specific treatments to individual patient genetic profiling will become possible. If truly effective, this should lead to an even earlier diagnosis for the 'high-risk' individual, ideally to more precise treatment interventions with improved response rates and hopefully reduced morbidity with minimal side effects.

It is hoped that the future will also see a structured and coordinated approach to developing multicentre, prospective randomised treatment trials. These trials need to investigate further the efficacy of potentially malignant disorder management, help improve the evidence base of our scientific literature, and perhaps most significantly of all develop new and innovative treatment strategies for our patients. Ultimately, it will only be by marshalling preventive and appropriately targeted early interventional strategies to effectively treat these potentially malignant disorders that we will see a reduction in the incidence of new cases of oral cancer, overall improvements in patient morbidity and mortality and then perhaps finally a halt to the impending threat of a worldwide oral cancer epidemic.

Index

Note: page numbers in *italics* refer to figures; those in **bold** refer to tables and boxes